Retina Atlas

Series Editors

Sandeep Saxena, Department of Ophthalmology
King George's Medical University
Lucknow, Uttar Pradesh, India

Richard F. Spaide, Vitreous Retina Macula Consultants of New York
New York, NY, USA

Eric H. Souied, Department of Ophthalmology
University Paris-Est Créteil
Créteil Cedex, France

Timothy Y. Y. Lai, Dept of Ophthalmology & Visual Sciences
Chinese University of Hong Kong
Hong Kong, Hong Kong

The 9-volume atlas covers validated and comprehensive information on retinal imaging, retinal vascular disorders, macular disorders, vitreoretinal surgical diseases, infectious and inflammatory disorders, retinal degenerations and dystrophies, pediatric retinal diseases, oncology, and trauma. This atlas with over 100 chapters is well supported with hundreds of high-quality images and text notes providing in-depth details and information in a well-organized manner.

The editors Sandeep Saxena (India), Richard F. Spaide (USA), Eric H. Souied (France) and Timothy Y. Y. Lai (Hong Kong), volume editors and contributing authors are reputed eye physicians in their field with vast clinical experience.

This series has a full dedicated volume on imaging and includes various imaging technologies like optical coherence tomography, fluorescein angiography, etc. It provides global perspective of vitreoretinal diseases extensively covering medical and surgical aspects of the disease. Uncommon retinal findings in diseases such as Dengue hemorrhagic fever, malaria etc. are also covered well.

Retina Atlas is a useful go-to series meant for ophthalmology residents, retina fellows, and retina specialists as well as general ophthalmologists.

Key Features

- Features coverage of retina in 9 volumes and more than hundred chapters enabling selective reading
- Covers full spectrum of retinal diseases and includes recent advances in imaging techniques
- Provides global perspective of vitreoretinal diseases for the first time covering extensively medical and surgical aspects of the disease
- Presents global expertise and knowledge of reputed experts working at high-volume centers of excellence

'Retina Atlas' series includes the following 9 Volumes:

1. Retinal Imaging
2. Retinal Vascular Disorders
3. Macular Disorders
4. Surgical Retina
5. Inflammatory and Infectious Ocular Disorders
6. Hereditary Chorioretinal Disorders
7. Pediatric Retinal Diseases
8. Ocular Oncology
9. Trauma and Miscellaneous Disorders in Retina

More information about this series at https://link.springer.com/bookseries/16451

R. V. Paul Chan
Editor

Pediatric Retinal Diseases

Springer

Editor
R. V. Paul Chan
Illinois Eye and Ear Infirmary
University of Illinois at Chicago
Chicago, IL, USA

ISSN 2662-5741 ISSN 2662-575X (electronic)
Retina Atlas
ISBN 978-981-19-1363-1 ISBN 978-981-19-1364-8 (eBook)
https://doi.org/10.1007/978-981-19-1364-8

This Springer imprint is published by the registered company Springer Nature Singapore Pte Ltd.
The registered company address is: 152 Beach Road, #21-01/04 Gateway East, Singapore 189721, Singapore

Contents

About the Editor

R. V. Paul Chan, MD, MSc is the Department Head and the John H. Panton, MD Professor of Ophthalmology at the Illinois Eye and Ear Infirmary, University of Illinois at Chicago (UIC). His clinical practice focuses on vitreoretinal surgery, with an expertise in pediatric retinal disease. Dr. Chan received his BA from the University of Pennsylvania, MD from the Temple University School of Medicine, MSc from Weill Cornell Medical College (WCMC), and MBA from the University of Chicago's Booth School of Business. After completing Ophthalmology residency at the New York-Presbyterian Hospital of WCMC, he went on to a Fellowship in Vitreoretinal Surgery at the Massachusetts Eye and Ear Infirmary at Harvard Medical School. Dr. Chan spent nine years on faculty at WCMC, as Director of the Retina Service and Vitreoretinal Fellowship, before moving to UIC. Dr. Chan previously served as the Vice Chair for both Clinical Affairs and Global Ophthalmology in the Department of Ophthalmology and Visual Sciences at UIC and is a global leader in pediatric blindness prevention and retinopathy of prematurity (ROP). His primary research interests focus on utilizing new technology and imaging techniques to better evaluate and manage children with retinal disease. He has authored over 180 peer reviewed articles and has received grant funding by the NIH, the NSF, and a number of charitable foundations. He is a core team member of the Imaging and Informatics for ROP (i-ROP) consortium and leads the Global Education Network for ROP (GEN-ROP), which is an international collaboration of investigators with expertise in neonatology, ophthalmology, biomedical informatics, international health, and medical education. Together, they have developed tele-education and telemedicine programs, and have established clinical, teaching, and research collaborations in Asia, Latin America, and Africa. Dr. Chan also serves as a consultant for programs sponsored by the United States Agency for International Development (USAID), Orbis International, and Helen Keller International (HKI). Dr. Chan is a leader in academic ophthalmology and organized medicine. He serves on the Board of Trustees for HKI, the Board of Trustees for Prevent Blindness America, the Executive Committee for the Pan-American Association of Ophthalmology (PAAO), and the Committee of Secretaries for the American Academy of Ophthalmology (AAO), where he is the Secretary for Global Alliances.

OCT Angiography for Pediatric Retinal Disease

1

J. Peter Campbell, Eric Nudleman, Sang Jin Kim, and Michael F. Chiang

Introduction

Optical coherence tomography angiography (OCTA) is an emerging imaging technology that is increasingly being used in retinal disease diagnosis and management. OCTA has relative advantages and disadvantages compared with standard fluorescein angiography (FA). It has the advantage of being able to produce three-dimensional angiographic images of the retina with capillary resolution without dye injection. However, the field of view is much smaller than FA, especially ultra-widefield FA, which has become commonly used in practice. Also, since angiographic flow is identified by repeat scans at the same point detecting relative differences in signal intensity due to the motion of red blood cells, it is sensitive to motion artifact, which has limited its use in patients with poor cooperation, such as young children. There have been a few reports using commercially available table-top OCTA devices to obtain images of children with retinal disease (de Carlo et al. 2015; Vinekar et al. 2016; Veronese et al. 2016). There are also several prototype swept source OCTA devices that have been reported for use in children, either in the operating room (Chen et al. 2017) or in clinic (Yang et al. 2017; Campbell et al. 2017a). The purpose of this chapter is to summarize the available literature and discuss the potential role for OCTA in the diagnosis of pediatric retinal disease in the future. An important question with any new imaging technology is whether it adds value to the clinical exam or standard of care diagnostic testing. For pediatric retinal disease, for the most part, this remains an important area of ongoing research.

J. P. Campbell
OHSU Eye Institute, Portland, OR, USA

E. Nudleman
UCSD Department of Ophthalmology, La Jolla, CA, USA

S. J. Kim
Samsung Medical Center Department of Ophthalmology, Seoul, Korea

M. F. Chiang (✉)
National Institutes of Health, Bethesda, MD, USA
e-mail: michael.chiang@nih.gov

OCTA in Pediatric Macular Disease

OCTA can diagnose the presence of choroidal neovascular membranes (CNV), which can lead to vision loss in a number of pediatric retinal diseases (Fig. 1.1) (Veronese et al. 2016). These cases are rare, but challenging both in terms of diagnosis by standard of care FA, and treatment with intravitreal injection. These evaluations, like many in pediatric retina, often require examination under anesthesia (EUA). However, recent evidence regarding the effects of anesthesia on the developing brain has resulted in resistance, from both parents and providers, to perform EUAs (Andropoulos and Greene 2017). Thus, in a cooperative child, the ability to rule in or out CNV without an FA and without an EUA would have immense practical importance.

OCTA in Pediatric Retinal Vascular Disease

The use of OCTA in adult retinal vascular disease, such as diabetic retinopathy (DR) and retinal vein occlusions, to quantifiably and objectively detect capillary injury that correlates with clinical disease severity has been rapidly expanding (Hwang et al. 2016). There has been some early intrigue in the use of OCTA in pediatric retinal vascular diseases such as retinopathy of prematurity (ROP), familial x-linked vitreoretinopathy (FEVR), incontinentia pigmenti (IP), sickle cell retinopathy (SCR), Coats disease and others. It is less clear how OCTA might replace the use of FA in these cases since the peripheral angiographic findings are so important to disease management, but there are at least three ways in which OCTA could add value in the diagnosis of these conditions. First, in DR, OCTA is demonstrating promise as an imaging method that can produce objective measurements of disease severity (e.g., total retinal of blood flow, flow void

R. V. P. Chan (ed.), *Pediatric Retinal Diseases*, Retina Atlas, https://doi.org/10.1007/978-981-19-1364-8_1

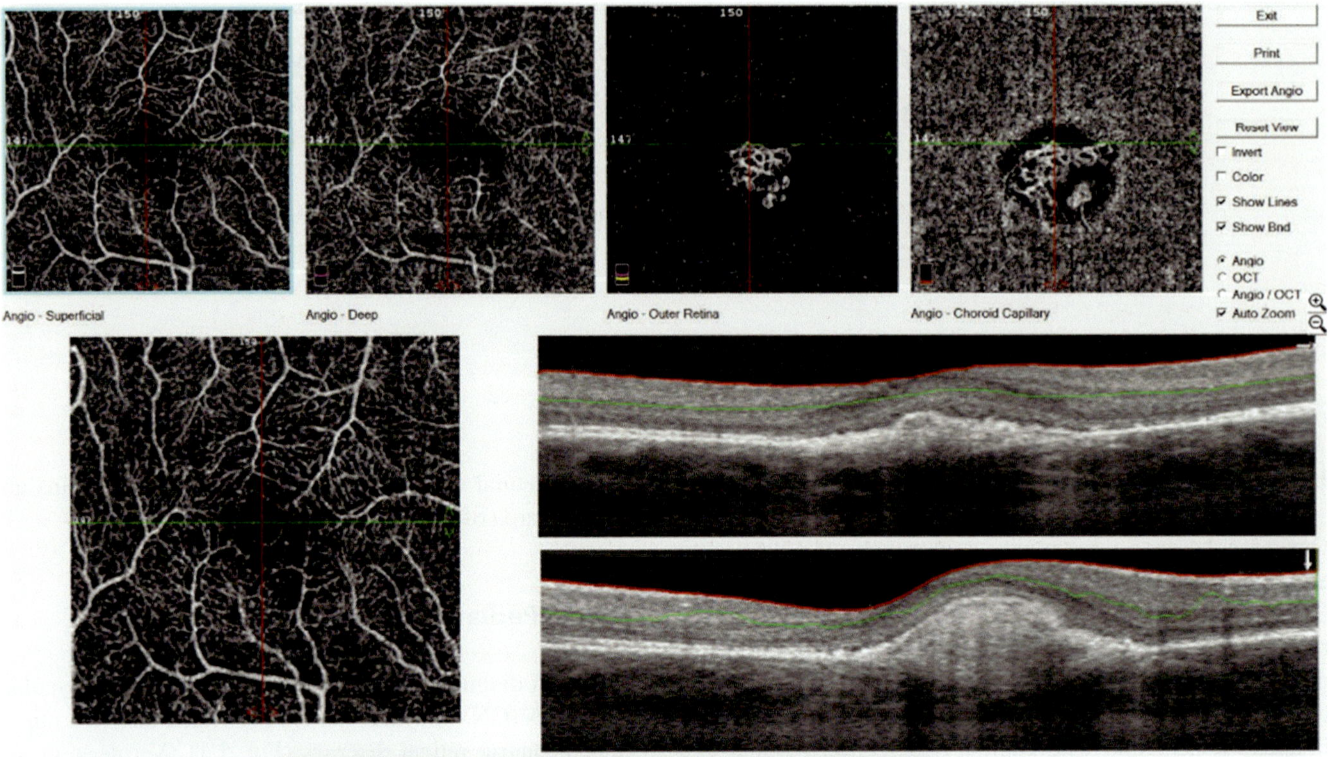

Fig. 1.1 Automated output from the Optovue Angiovue OCTA demonstrating flow in the outer retinal space due to a choroidal neovascular membrane in a 12 year old with Best disease

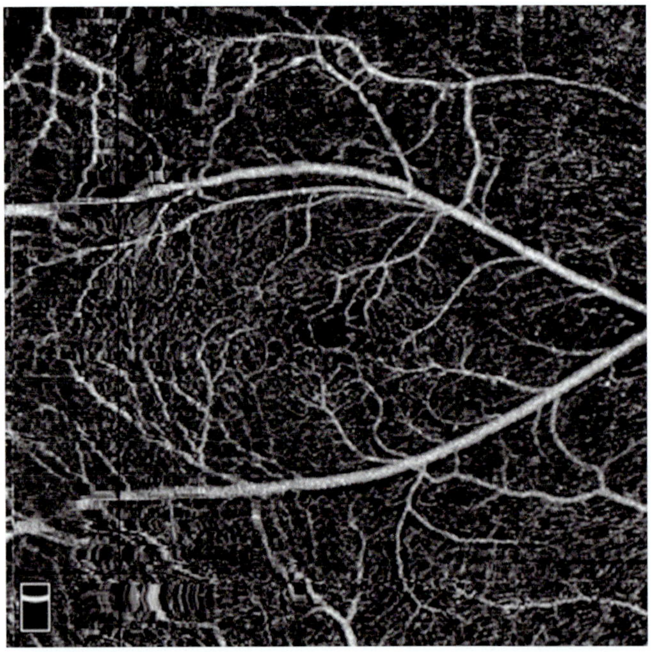

Fig. 1.2 OCTA image of a patient with Familial Exudative Vitreoretinopathy demonstrating straightening of the vascular arcades

areas, and vessel density) that correlate with clinical disease severity, and the same could be true in pediatric retinal vascular diseases such as FEVR (Fig. 1.2), IP, and SCR.

Second, OCTA is able to uniquely visualize not only the superficial vascular plexuses of the retina (in the nerve fiber layer and ganglion cell layer), but also the deeper vascular plexuses, typically called the intermediate and deep capillary plexuses (ICP and DCP), which are not well visualized by FA (Weinhaus et al. 1995). In adults, we are learning more about the unique role these capillary plexuses play in certain vascular conditions, and the same may be true in pediatric retinal disease (Sarraf et al. 2013; Campbell et al. 2017b). For example, animal models of FEVR suggest that the ICP and DCP fail to develop normally due to mutations in the Wnt signaling pathway, (Gilmour: 2014kd) however, this hypothesis has not yet been demonstrated in vivo in humans.

Third, foveal development and perfusion are critical to vision, and both can be abnormal in these conditions. In severe ROP, we know from cross-sectional studies using OCTA in older children that the foveal avascular zone (FAZ) is incompletely developed in many cases (Vinekar et al. 2016). (Falavarjani et al. 2017bw) In IP, progressive nonperfusion can lead to atrophy of a previously structurally normal fovea and foveal avascular zone, which can be seen by OCTA. Since OCTA can be obtained without the risk of serial intravenous injection, it provides the potential to better understand the pathophysiology of these conditions and in theory detect disease progression at an earlier state (as in Fig. 1.3).

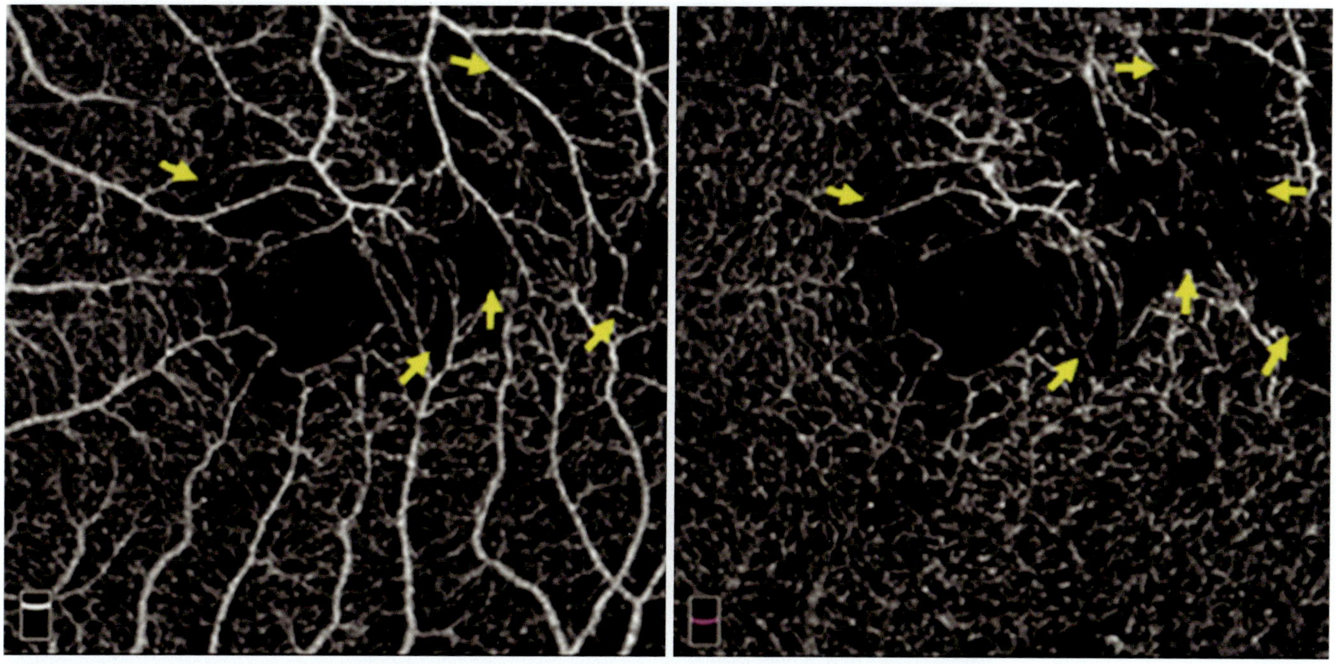

Fig. 1.3 OCTA image of a 17-year-old with sickle cell retinopathy demonstrating reduced vessel density (arrows) in both the superficial (left) and more significantly in the deep (right) segmentations on the Optovue Angiovue system (images courtesy of Adrienne Scott, MD, Wilmer Eye Institute)

Portable OCTA

One of the main limitations with the widespread application and investigation of this technology in pediatric retinal disease is the limitations of currently available technology. All of the commercially available devices are table mounted, designed for adult heads, and require cooperation for fixation for at least a few seconds per scan. Thus, though older children with good vision may be able to use these devices, the technology has been inaccessible for young children or those without the ability to fixate. Investigators at Duke University have developed a microscope mounted swept source (SS) OCTA and demonstrate the use of intraoperative OCTA for patients undergoing examinations under anesthesia or surgery (Chen et al. 2017). However, there has not been technology available for use in outpatients or neonates in the intensive care unit with ROP. To address this need, we have developed a portable SS-OCTA device at Oregon Health & Science University (OHSU) Casey Eye Institute (Yang et al. 2017; Campbell et al. 2017a). We have successfully obtained images in patients sedated and non-sedated with ROP, IP, Coats, FEVR and a variety of less common pediatric retinal conditions (Figs. 1.4 and 1.5). In the same way that portable OCT technology has improved our understanding of structural retinal changes in these conditions (Lee et al. 2016), OCTA may provide added insight into the pathophysiology of these conditions.

One of the most interesting potential applications of this technology is the monitoring of normal retinal vascular development following premature birth. In theory, serial OCTA could help illuminate the fundamental processes of angiogenesis and vasculogenesis, and the sequence of microvascular changes that lead to the development of the FAZ. Much of our understanding of ROP physiology comes from *ex vivo* examination of animal models of oxygen-induced retinopathy (OIR), which are imperfect models for a number of reasons including the animals are not preterm, the pathophysiology often does not recapitulate typical ROP and thus has unclear relevance to anatomic biomarkers predictive of clinically significant disease. Finally, the OIR rodent models do not have a FAZ and thus the model cannot facilitate studies determining the factors responsible for the maldevelopment of the FAZ, which has clinically relevant implications for vision. Thus, serial examination of preterm babies using OCTA may improve not only our understanding of ROP pathophysiology, but may also illuminate fundamental principles of retinal angiogenesis. Much of this remains to be proven, and will be greatly facilitated by the availability of commercially available portable OCTA.

Conclusion

OCTA has the potential to change the way adults with macular disease are diagnosed and managed, and the same may be true in children with pediatric retinal disease. Over the next few years, as the technology becomes faster, less

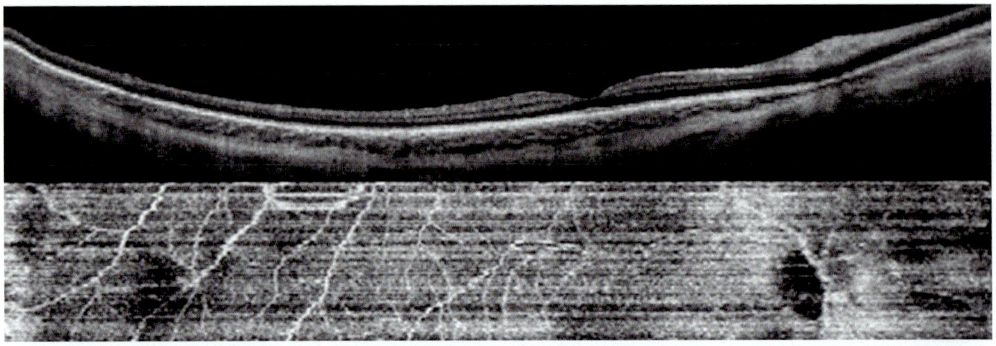

Fig. 1.4 Prototype widefield swept source OCT (top) and OCTA (bottom) image of a neonate obtained during ROP screening in the neonatal intensive care unit demonstrating perfusion into zone 2

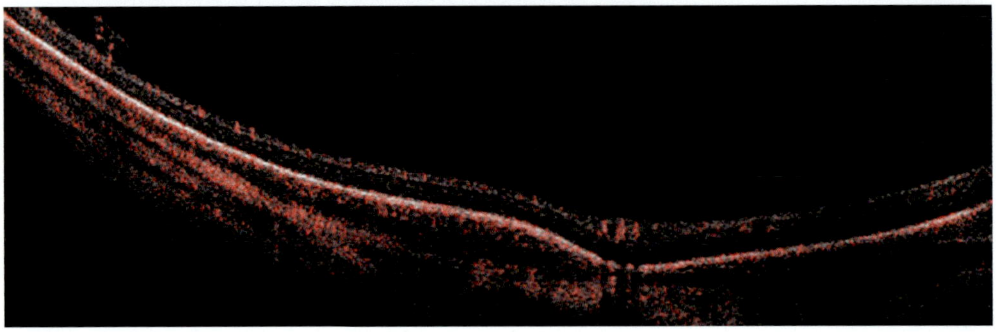

Fig. 1.5 Cross-sectional OCT/OCTA image obtained using a prototype swept source OCTA demonstrating flow (in red) above the internal limiting membrane (extraretinal neovascularization) in a preterm infant undergoing ROP screening

expensive, and more widely available, we will be seeing increasing numbers of reports of the use of OCTA in the pediatric population. As clinicians, our job will be to evaluate the clinical utility of this technology and demonstrate the added value it may provide to the care of children with the goals of: (1) reducing the need for examinations under anesthesia, (2) improving our fundamental understanding of disease pathophysiology which may lead to improved therapeutic interventions, and (3) improving outcomes, in the future.

References

Andropoulos DB, Greene MF. Anesthesia and developing brains — implications of the FDA warning. N Engl J Med. 2017;376(10):905–7. https://doi.org/10.1056/NEJMp1700196.

Campbell JP, Nudleman E, Yang J, et al. Handheld optical coherence tomography angiography and ultra-wide-field optical coherence tomography in retinopathy of prematurity. JAMA Ophthalmol. 2017a;135(9):977–81. https://doi.org/10.1001/jamaophthalmol.2017.2481.

Campbell JP, Zhang M, Hwang TS, et al. Detailed vascular anatomy of the human retina by projection-resolved optical coherence tomography angiography. Sci Rep. 2017b;7:42201. https://doi.org/10.1038/srep42201.

Chen X, Viehland C, Carrasco-Zevallos OM, et al. Microscope-integrated optical coherence tomography angiography in the operating room in young children with retinal vascular disease. JAMA Ophthalmol. 2017:1–4. https://doi.org/10.1001/jamaophthalmol.2017.0422&utm_campaign=articlePDF%26utm_medium=articlePDFlink%26utm_source=articlePDF%26utm_content=jamaophthalmol.2017.0422.

Falavarjani KG, Iafe NA, Velez FG, Schwartz SD, Sadda SR, Sarraf D, Tsui I. Optical coherence tomography angiography of the fovea in children born preterm. Retina. 2017;37(12):2289–94. https://doi.org/10.1097/IAE.0000000000001471. PMID: 28098735.

de Carlo TE, Romano A, Waheed NK, Duker JS. A review of optical coherence tomography angiography (OCTA). Int J Retina Vitreous. 2015;1(1):1. https://doi.org/10.1186/s40942-015-0005-8.

Gilmour DF. Familial exudative vitreoretinopathy and related retinopathies. Eye (Lond). 2015;29(1):1–14. https://doi.org/10.1038/eye.2014.70. Epub 2014 Oct 17. PMID: 25323851; PMCID: PMC4289842.

Hwang TS, Gao SS, Liu L, et al. Automated quantification of capillary nonperfusion using optical coherence tomography angiography in diabetic retinopathy. JAMA Ophthalmol. 2016;134(4):367–73. https://doi.org/10.1001/jamaophthalmol.2015.5658.

Lee H, Proudlock FA, Gottlob I. Pediatric optical coherence tomography in clinical practice-recent progress. Invest Ophthalmol Vis Sci. 2016;57(9):OCT69–79. https://doi.org/10.1167/iovs.15-18825.

Sarraf D, Rahimy E, Fawzi AA, et al. Paracentral acute middle maculopathy: a new variant of acute macular neuroretinopathy associated with retinal capillary ischemia. JAMA Ophthalmol. 2013;131(10):1275–87. https://doi.org/10.1001/jamaophthalmol.2013.4056.

Veronese C, Maiolo C, Huang D, et al. Optical coherence tomography angiography in pediatric choroidal neovascularization. Am J Ophthalmol Case Rep. 2016;2:37–40. https://doi.org/10.1016/j.ajoc.2016.03.009.

Vinekar A, Chidambara L, Jayadev C, Sivakumar M, Webers CAB, Shetty B. Monitoring neovascularization in aggressive posterior retinopathy of prematurity using optical coherence tomography angiography. J AAPOS. 2016;20(3):271–4. https://doi.org/10.1016/j.jaapos.2016.01.013.

Weinhaus RS, Burke JM, Delori FC, Snodderly DM. Comparison of fluorescein angiography with microvascular anatomy of macaque retinas. Exp Eye Res. 1995;61(1):1–16.

Yang J, Liu L, Campbell JP, Huang D, Liu G. Handheld optical coherence tomography angiography. Biomed Opt Express. 2017;8(4):2287–14. https://doi.org/10.1364/BOE.8.002287.

Retinopathy of Prematurity

2

Daniel Oh, Ru-Ik Chee, Andrew Tsai, Gavin Tan, Wei-Chi Wu, and R. V. Paul Chan

Introduction

Retinopathy of prematurity is a vasoproliferative disease of the retina that affects premature infants to varying degrees. Almost 3.9 million infants are born in the USA, of which about 10% are born premature. Of those infants who are born premature, about 14,000–16,000 are affected to some degree of ROP (National Eye Institute). In most cases, the disease improves without treatment and has no permanent sequelae; however, infants with more severe disease may require medical or surgical intervention. In all, about 400–600 infants each year in the USA become legally blind from ROP (National Eye Institute).

Retinopathy of prematurity, once termed retrolental fibroplasia, was described by Theodore Terry in 1942 (Terry 1942). Gray membranes with blood vessels behind the pupil of neonates were observed (Phelps 1992). Three distinct epidemics have been described globally since Terry's description of retinopathy of prematurity (Gilbert 2008). The first epidemic in the 1940s and 1950s primarily affected premature babies in the USA and Western Europe where unmonitored supplemental oxygen was the driving risk factor (Gilbert 2008). A second epidemic began in the 1970s in industrialized countries as a consequence of higher survival rates in premature babies with even lower birth weights and earlier gestational ages from increased use of intensive neonatal care units (Gilbert 2008). A third epidemic is believed to have occurred in the 1990s now mostly in middle-income countries from access to neonatal intensive care units in these countries and risk factors such as higher rates of teen pregnancy (Gilbert 2008; Shah et al. 2009). There are also phenotypic variations as ROP from these developing regions tends to develop in more mature and larger babies (Quinn 2016). As we transition toward a potential fourth epidemic of ROP from widespread adoption of higher oxygen saturations (shift from 88–92% to 92–95%) in preterm infants, we are reminded of the persistent clinical challenges that remain with the management of pediatric retinal conditions and ROP (Cayabyab and Ramanathan 2016).

Pathogenesis

Retinopathy of prematurity has been closely tied with fetal oxygen supply as evidenced by the first epidemic of ROP (Cavallaro et al. 2014). In the human fetus, retinal blood vessels begin to develop during the fourth month of gestation (Smith 2004). The pathogenesis of ROP is divided into two phases. In the first phase, there is a cessation of normal retinal vascular development, and as the infant matures, the nonvascularized retina continues to have increased metabolic demands leading to increasing hypoxia (Smith 2004). In the second phase, there is retinal neovascularization and occurs at 34 weeks' postmenstrual age (Ashton et al. 1954). Neovascularization occurs as vascular endothelial growth factor (VEGF) is increasingly expressed due to ischemia. Neovascularization is often described as a wave of physiologic hypoxia in that new blood vessels grow toward the VEGF stimulus, and as hypoxia is dampened by vascular oxygen, the wave propagates forward (Stone et al. 1995). If unchecked, retinal neovascularization progresses into a cicatricial phase which can result in macular dragging, vitreoretinal lens adhesions, and retinal detachment (Agarwal and Jalali 2018). Mouse models have shown that specifically inhibiting VEGF ceases the neovascular response, indicating that while other growth factors and cytokines are involved in hypoxia signaling vascularization, VEGF is critical in this

D. Oh · R.-I. Chee · R. V. P. Chan (✉)
Department of Ophthalmology and Visual Sciences, Illinois Eye and Ear Infirmary, University of Illinois at Chicago, Chicago, IL, USA
e-mail: rvpchan@uic.edu

A. Tsai · G. Tan
Singapore National Eye Center, Ophthalmology and Visual Sciences, Duke-NUS Medical School, National University of Singapore, Singapore, Singapore

W.-C. Wu
Chang Gung Memorial Hospital, Taoyuan, Taiwan

R. V. P. Chan (ed.), *Pediatric Retinal Diseases*, Retina Atlas, https://doi.org/10.1007/978-981-19-1364-8_2

process (Smith 2004). It is important to note that apart from being an important angiogenic factor during embryonic vascular development, VEGF also plays an important role in the development of the kidney, lungs, and skeletal and hematopoietic systems (Chan-Ling et al. 2018).

Aside from VEGF, other signaling molecules have been investigated closely. In both normal mice treated with somatostatin decreasing growth hormone and transgenic mice expressing GH-receptor antagonist, neovascularization in phase II of ROP has been observed (Smith 2004). Specifically, GH inhibition of neovascularization is through IGF-1 as administering IGF-1 systemically was found to restore neovascularization in mice (Smith 2004). An IGF-1 antagonist was used to suppress neovascularization independent of VEGF (Smith). In addition, IGF-1 has been described as a factor expressed independent of hypoxia. In premature infants, mean IFT-1 levels were found to be significantly lower with higher ROP stages than those without ROP (Smith 2004).

The role of HIF-1a, a heterodimer with the a-subunit regulated by hypoxia and the b-subunit constitutively expressed, has also been investigated. Reduced HIF-1a levels reduce VEGF expression and induce the regression of retinal vessels, critical for phase I of ROP (Cavallaro et al. 2014). However, it increases in phase II ROP, parallel to VEGF, leading to neovascularization (Cavallaro et al. 2014). Other signaling molecules that have been explored include nitric oxide (NO), placental growth factor (PIGF), adenosine, apelin, and b-adrenergic receptors (Cavallaro et al. 2014). Such signaling molecules have been linked to each other, oxygen levels, and angiogenesis.

Clinical Classification and Features

International Classification of ROP: Zones, Stages, Plus, APROP

The International Classification of Retinopathy of Prematurity (ICROP) was published in two parts: the first in 1984 and then expanded in 1987 (Prematurity ICftCoRo 2005). Currently, additional revisions to ICROP are underway and updates will be presented in the near future. The original ICROP took into account the location of retinal involvement, the extent of retinal involvement by clock hour, the stage or severity of retinopathy, and the presence or absence of dilated and tortuous posterior pole vessels (plus disease) (Fig. 2.1).

The location of disease was described as three concentric zones, each centered on the optic disc rather than the macula. This was selected because the normal retinal vessels proceed from the center of the optic disc toward the ora serrata (Prematurity ICftCoRo 2005). Zone I consists of a circle and is the innermost zone which extends from the center of the optic disc to twice the distance from the center of the optic disc to the fovea. Zone II consists of the area that extends from the edge of zone I to the nasal ora serrata. Zone III is the remaining portion of the retina that is anterior to zone II, thus completing the temporal retina.

The stage of severity of disease is explained by qualitative findings on funduscopic examination. Stage 1 is characterized by a thin but definite demarcation line separating the avascular retina anteriorly from the vascularized retina posteriorly (Prematurity ICftCoRo 2005). There is abnormal vessels leading up to the demarcation line which itself is often white and flat, lying in the plane of the retina (Prematurity ICftCoRo 2005). Stage 2 is characterized by a ridge, arising from the demarcation line, but now possessing a height and width extending above the plane of the retina (Fig. 2.2).

The ridge itself may become pink and vessels may enter the ridge posteriorly (Prematurity ICftCoRo 2005). Areas of neovascular tissue may be seen posterior to the ridge structure (Prematurity ICftCoRo 2005). Stage 3 is defined by extraretinal fibrovascular proliferation or neovascularization extending from the ridge into the vitreous (Fig. 2.3).

Stage 4 is divided into extrafoveal (stage 4A) and foveal (stage 4B) partial retinal detachments (ICROP) (Fig. 2.4). The extent of the retinal detachment is dependent on the extent of fibrovascular involvement. The fibrous tissue can continue to contract leading to larger tractional retinal detachments.

Finally, stage 5 is characterized by a total retinal detachment, while usually tractional, they may also be exudative (Prematurity ICftCoRo 2005). In severe cases, the retinal detachment can become funnel-shaped.

The presence of findings including increased venous dilatation and arteriolar tortuosity in at least two quadrants of the eye has been isolated as an additional risk of rapidly progressing ROP. Milder forms of these vascular abnormalities are referred to as pre-plus disease while more severe forms are termed plus disease. Pre-plus disease (Fig. 2.5) may be predictive of progression of disease necessitating laser treatment (Wallace et al. 2011).

A rapidly progressing severe form of ROP termed aggressive posterior ROP or AP-ROP has been described and is a form of ROP, which, if untreated, can progress quickly to stage 5 ROP. It is most commonly observed in zone I but may occur in posterior zone II. AP-ROP is characterized by its posterior location, prominence of plus disease usually manifest by vascular abnormalities in all four quadrants out of proportion with the peripheral retinopathy. Usually, AP-ROP does not progress through the classic stages 1–3 and may first appear as a small flat area of neovascularization at the junction between vascularized and non-vascularized retina, allowing it to be missed (Prematurity ICftCoRo 2005).

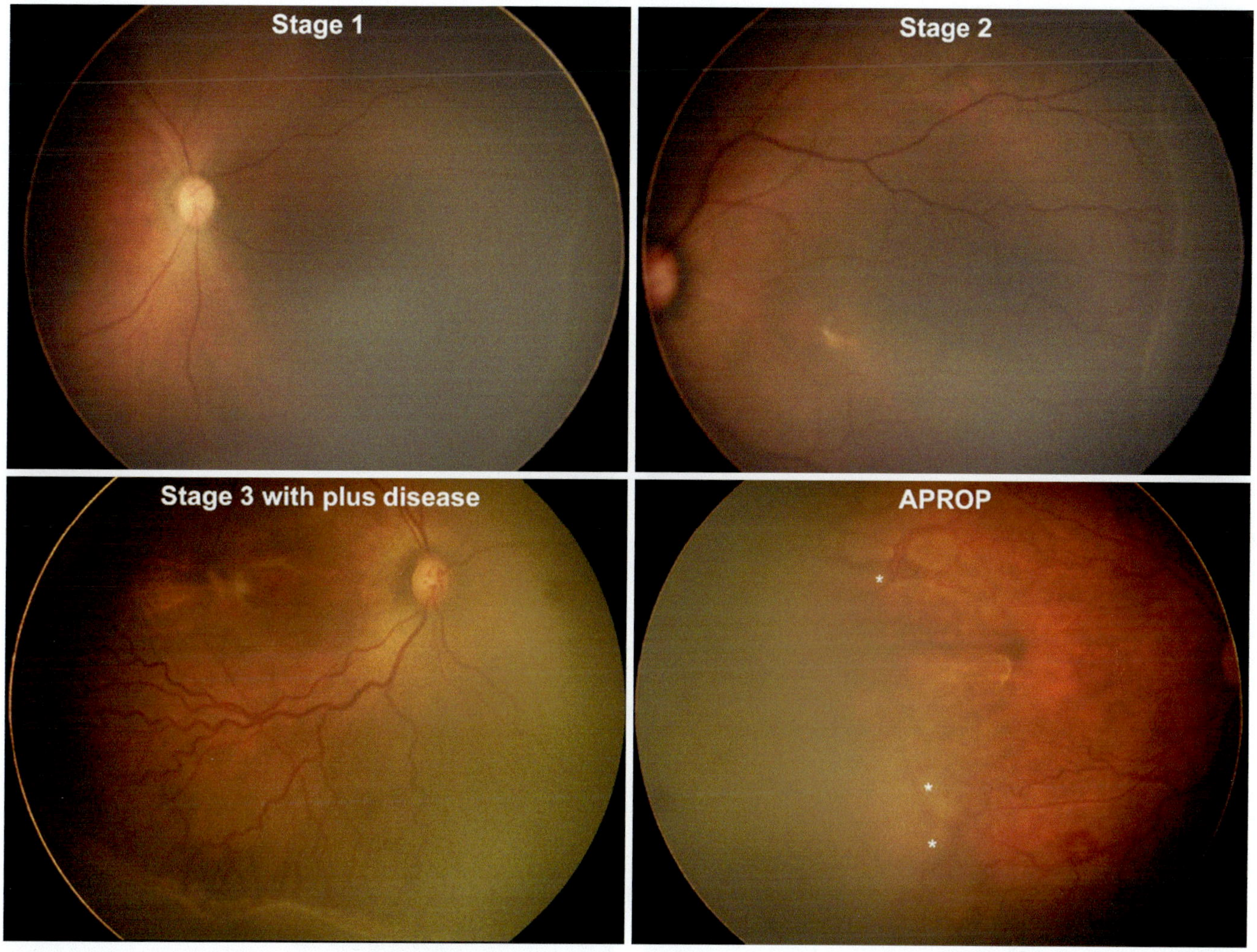

Fig. 2.1 RetCam images of ROP stages, plus disease, and aggressive posterior ROP

The Early Treatment for Retinopathy of Prematurity (ETROP) study distinguished type 1 and type 2 disease where treatment is necessary for type 1 ROP. Type 1 ROP was defined as zone I with any stage and plus disease, zone I with stage 3 without plus disease, and zone II, stage 2 or 3 with plus disease. Type 2 ROP which does not necessarily require treatment was defined as zone I, stage 1 or 2 without plus disease, and zone II, stage without plus disease (Good and Group ETfRoPC 2004).

Other Features

Other findings in retinopathy of prematurity include macular dragging, often associated with poor vision and caused by significant levels of traction from fibrovascular membranes, temporal vessel straightening, and vitreous hemorrhage (Gupta et al. 2016). Narrowing of the angle of retinal vessels at the juxtapapillary entrance, retinal pigmentary changes, and macular ectopy have also been observed (Cerman et al. 2016).

Screening

Screening Criteria

A joint statement from the American Academy of Pediatrics (AAP), American Academy of Ophthalmology (AAO), and the American Association for Pediatric Ophthalmology and Strabismus (AAPOS) introduced recommendations for infants with a birth weight of less than or equal to 1500 g or gestational age of 30 weeks or less to be screened by binocular indirect ophthalmoscopy with a lid speculum and scleral depression (AAP). Infants of birth weight between 1500 and 2000 g or gestational age >30 weeks with an unstable clinical course, including those requiring cardiorespiratory support and who are at high risk as determined by the pediatrician or neonatologist, also qualify for screening (AAP). However, in low- or middle-income countries, ROP may occur in infants with larger birth weight and older gestational age. As such, screening criteria may vary according to the population

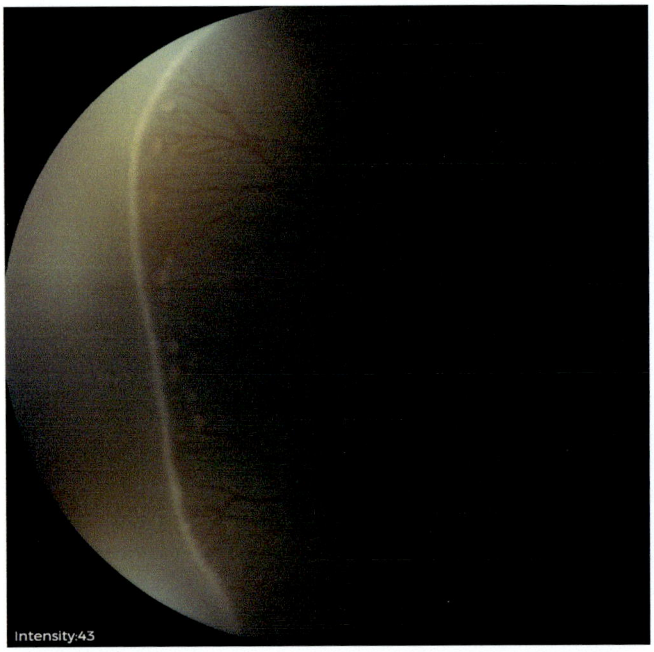

Fig. 2.2 RetCam image of stage 2 ROP with isolated neovascular tufts "popcorn"

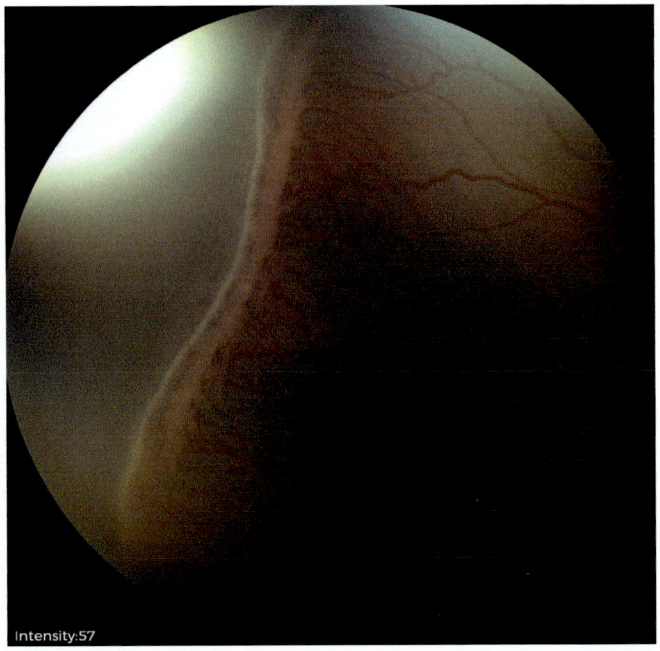

Fig. 2.3 RetCam image of stage 3 ROP

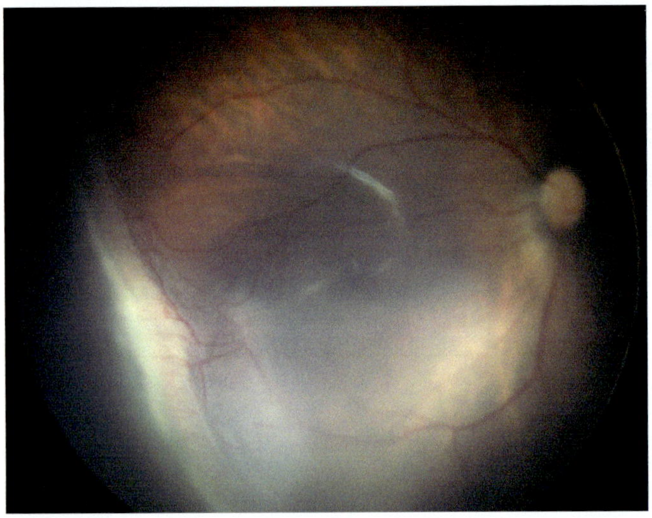

Fig. 2.4 RetCam image of stage 4A retinal detachment

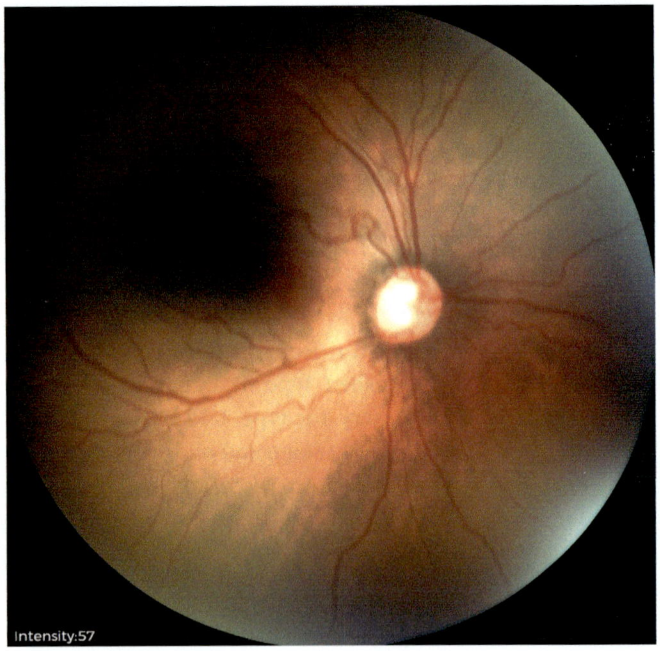

Fig. 2.5 RetCam image of pre-plus disease

of premature infants being cared for in various countries (Quinn 2016).

Follow-up exams of 1 week, 1–2 weeks, 2 weeks, and 2–3 week intervals have been suggested.

1 week or less follow-up has been suggested for immature vascularization in zone I, immature retina extending into posterior zone II near the boundary of zone I, stage 1 or 2 ROP: zone I, stage 3 ROP: zone II, or the presence or suspected presence of AP-ROP.

1- to 2-week follow-up has been suggested for immature vascularization in posterior zone II, stage 2 ROP: zone II, and regressing ROP: zone I.

2-week follow-up has been suggested for stage 1 ROP: zone II, immature vascularization: zone II—no ROP, and regression ROP: zone II.

2- to 3-week follow-up has been suggested for stage 1 or 2 ROP: zone III, regression ROP: zone III.

Termination of Screening Criteria

Termination of exams has been suggested based on age and retinal findings. The joint statement by AAP, AAO, and AAPOS includes the termination of exams based on zone III retinal vascularization attained without previous zone I or II ROP, full retinal vascularization near the ora serrata for 360 degrees, postmenstrual age of 50 weeks and no pre-threshold disease, or regression of ROP.

Future Screening Criteria

Newer predictors of ROP have been proposed with various neonatal scoring systems to help identify neonates at higher risk of developing severe ROP (Fortes Filho et al. 2009; Zepeda-Romero et al. 2012; Binenbaum et al. 2018; Löfqvist et al. 2009; Aydemir et al. 2011; Pérez-Muñuzuri et al. 2010; Pieh et al. 2010; Piyasena et al. 2014; Eckert et al. 2012).

Telemedicine

While clinical examination of patients through indirect ophthalmoscopy is the gold standard by which ROP is diagnosed, there is a shortage of experts needed for ROP examinations (Chee et al. 2018). Consequently, imaging tools have been increasingly used such that diagnoses can be made via telecommunication, particularly in underserved regions and countries. While similar approaches have been explored in other medical specialties, much is yet to be understood regarding the validity, risks, cost, and feasibility across clinical sites for such an approach in ROP diagnosis and management. In 2012, the American Academy of Ophthalmology Ophthalmic Technology Assessment Committee (OTAC) reported high accuracy (over 90% sensitivity) for the detection of clinically significant ROP with wide-angle retinal photography (Chiang et al. 2012). In addition, a report in 2015 by the American Academy of Pediatrics and the American Academy of Ophthalmology examined the implementation of telemedicine for ROP, again indicating the high accuracy for detection of clinically significant ROP with wide-angle digital photography (Silva et al. 2011).

Ongoing screening programs have been established in several countries, including low- and middle-income countries (Fijalkowski et al. 2013). However, it has yet to be observed whether screening criteria are consistent across countries given varying resources and demographics across countries. Consequently, efforts to challenge existing screening guidelines or establish new ones are in effect.

The quality of images used for telemedicine understandably has a critical impact in its success. The RetCam (Clarity Medical Systems, Inc., Pleasanton, CA), a mydriatic wide-field fundus imaging system achieving a 130 degree field of view, has been adopted by neonatal intensive care units (NICUs) across the USA (Chee et al. 2018). Other pediatric retinal imaging systems include PanoCam LT (Visunex Medical Systems, Fremont, CA) and 3nethra neo (Forus Health, Bangalore, India) systems (Chee et al. 2018). Optomap (Optos plc, Dunfermline, Scotland); a non-contact, non-mydriatic ultra-wide-field imaging system achieving a 200-degree field of view has also been explored as an alternative imaging tool in infants, although it has not yet been widely adopted for retinal imaging for ROP.

Telemedicine is particularly suited to diseases such as ROP where its prevalence is high in areas where access to skilled ophthalmologists and resources is lowest. However, establishing such programs continues to be challenging, especially with high levels of initial investment needed for imaging systems and personnel (Chee et al. 2018). Nevertheless, telemedicine for ROP has been shown to be cost-effective (Jackson et al. 2008). Other directions for the future of ROP telemedicine include the increasing use of fluorescein angiography in the evaluation of pediatric patients, imaging montaging software programs for increasing the field of view on a single image, and artificial intelligence in conjunction with ROP expert interpretation (Chee et al. 2018).

Management

Observation

Large studies including the Cryotherapy for ROP (CRYO-ROP) in 1988 and the Early Treatment for ROP (ETROP) in 2004 have set criteria for treating ROP. The majority (90%) of patients with ROP only require observation, with spontaneous resolution of disease. Only 10% of patients with ROP eventually require intervention based on treatment criteria (Good and Group ETfRoPC 2004).

Cryotherapy

The CRYO-ROP Study evaluated the effects of retinal cryoablation in infants with retinopathy of prematurity carried out in 23 centers across the USA (Group CfRoPC 2001).

Prior to CRYO-ROP, case series in the 1970s and 1980s supported peripheral retinal ablation prior to the development of fibrovascular membranes or retinal detachments (Nagata et al. 1982). CRYO-ROP established that treating immature avascular retina for threshold disease, five or more contiguous or eight total clock hours of stage 3 ROP in zones I or II with plus disease, improved outcomes. After 15 years, a decrease of more than 40% in structural outcomes and a decrease in 30% in unfavorable visual acuity outcomes were observed (Palmer).

Laser Photocoagulation

In 2004, ETROP specified that high-risk pre-threshold ROP or type 1 ROP, while not meeting threshold criteria, deserved treatment (Good). Treating high-risk pre-threshold ROP reduced unfavorable structural outcomes from 15.6% to 9.0% and unfavorable visual acuity outcomes from 19.8% to 14.3% (Good and Group ETfRoPC 2004). The pattern of laser should be near confluent to confluent covering the avascular retina from the ridge to the ora serrata. Skip areas can lead to treatment failure as avascular retina can continue to produce VEGF (Rezai et al. 2005).

Additionally, diode laser photocoagulation therapy, compared to cryoablation, had lower rates of eyelid and conjunctival complications (McNamara et al. 1992). In one study after 7 years, the mean visual acuity was 20/33 after laser photocoagulation and after cryoablation 20/133 with statistical significance (Shalev et al. 2001). Compared to cryotherapy, laser photocoagulation has also been shown to be associated with lower rates of myopia (Connolly et al. 2002).

Treatment Earlier Than Type 1

Treatment may be beneficial for infants with less than type 1 ROP (Gupta et al. 2016). In a multicenter retrospective review, 9.5% of eyes were treated with less than type 1 ROP given one or more of the following indications: active ROP with the fellow eye being treated for type 1 ROP, concerning structural changes including tangential traction with temporal vessel straightening concerning macular dragging, thick stage 3 membranes with anteroposterior traction concerning progression to stage 4 ROP, persistent ROP at an advanced postmenstrual age, and vitreous hemorrhage (Gupta et al. 2016). The role of individual clinical judgment in situations outside of evidenced-based treatment guidelines is emphasized in the study.

Anti-VEGF

Intravitreal anti-VEGF pharmacotherapy has been considered as an alternative treatment for retinopathy of prematurity. Currently, there is limited level I evidence for the use of anti-VEGF (Sankar et al. 2018). However, anti-VEGF treatment has been reported to include faster regression of ROP, lower risk of myopia, less stress on the infant, and less time needed for treatment administration (Mintz-Hittner et al. 2016; VanderVeen and Cataltepe 2019). Practically, it can be useful for zone I disease, unstable infants, and those in whom general anesthesia is contraindicated.

Numerous studies have investigated the safety and effectiveness of anti-VEGF for the treatment of ROP (VanderVeen and Cataltepe 2019; Mintz-Hittner et al. 2011; Zhang et al. 2017; Autrata et al. 2012; Mueller et al. 2017; Gunay et al. 2017).

There are, however, concerns of systemic safety in the use of intravitreal anti-VEGF, and it has been found that serum VEGF can be suppressed up to 2 months. VEGF is important for organogenesis and neurodevelopment in particular (Wu et al. 2015). The long-term effect of anti-VEGF on neurodevelopment has also yet to be determined, with studies yielding conflicting results (Wu and Wu 2018).

There are ongoing studies on lower doses on anti-VEGF to reduce the risk of systemic toxicity (Wallace et al. 2017), and newer agents in the pipeline such as aflibercept are being evaluated (CLINICALTrials.gov NCT04004208).

Vitreoretinal Surgery

Surgical options are considered for stage 4 (partial retinal detachment) and stage 5 (total retinal detachment) ROP. These options include vitrectomy with or without scleral buckling. Lensectomy may also be considered to improve access to the retina and maneuvering to reach anterior membranes (Shapiro et al. 2006). Amblyopia should be considered when removing the lens, specifically the contralateral fovea. Other complications of vitrectomy include cataracts, corneal opacity, glaucoma, and strabismus (Choi et al. 2012).

In general, the prognosis after ROP surgery is relatively poor for stage 5 ROP. A significant number of children subsequently develop significant neurological impairment, which further impairs visual function.

Follow-Up and Long-Term Effects After Regression

Refractive Error

Refractive error after cryotherapy, laser treatment, and anti-VEGF have been reported. In 2013, one study compared bevacizumab with laser photocoagulation and observed less myopia in eyes treated with bevacizumab compared to laser (Harder et al. 2013). In another study in 2015, less myopia was also observed with bevacizumab but only for eyes treated with zone II ROP and not zone I ROP (Hwang et al. 2015). Another 2015 study showed increased myopia in eyes treated with laser but was not significant (Isaac et al. 2015). Zone I ROP was found to be associated with myopia regardless of treatment choice in another study (Gunay et al. 2017).

Other Ocular Abnormalities

Lid edema, periorbital swelling, retinal hemorrhages, conjunctival tears, and conjunctival hematomas have all been reported after treatment with cryotherapy. Less commonly, scleral rupture may also occur with cryotherapy (Flynn and Tasman 1992). The following have been seen with laser photocoagulation: corneal haze from epithelial edema, miotic pupils, hyphemas, iris burns, and posterior retinal burns (Flynn and Tasman 1992). Less commonly, vitreous hemorrhage, inflammation and hypopyon, and rhegmatogenous retinal detachments have been reported to be associated with laser photocoagulation (Flynn and Tasman 1992).

Other Systemic Abnormalities

While systemic complications are not commonly associated with cryotherapy, anesthesia that may be necessary to administer treatment is associated with bradycardia, arrhythmia, and respiratory arrest. With laser photocoagulation, apnea and bradycardia have been reported (Spiegel and Lisa 2006). Anti-VEGF may diffuse into the systemic circulation and potentially cause toxicity. It has been found that serum suppression of VEGF was more pronounced for bevacizumab when compared to ranibizumab and aflibercept (Huang et al. 2018; Wu et al. 2017).

Importantly, several studies have looked at adverse neurodevelopmental effects of ROP treatment with anti-VEGF (Lien et al. 2016; Morin et al. 2016; Araz-Ersan et al. 2015).

Conclusion

Retinopathy of prematurity is a disease that has presented in different epidemics historically. Treatment of ROP has concurrently evolved over the years, traditionally with the use of cryotherapy and laser photocoagulation. The management paradigm in ROP continues to evolve with the development of new pharmacotherapeutics, retinal imaging technologies, telemedicine systems, computer-based image analysis, adoption of deep learning technology, and continued microsurgical advances. As new evidence emerges, the guidelines for the treatment of ROP may likewise be further honed, requiring practitioners to remain updated.

References

Agarwal K, Jalali S. Classification of retinopathy of prematurity: from then till now. Commun Eye Health. 2018;31(101):S4–7.

Araz-Ersan B, Kir N, Tuncer S, et al. Preliminary anatomical and neurodevelopmental outcomes of intravitreal bevacizumab as adjunctive treatment for retinopathy of prematurity. Curr Eye Res. 2015;40(6):585–91. https://doi.org/10.3109/02713683.2014.941070.

Ashton N, Ward B, Serpell G. Effect of oxygen on developing retinal vessels with particular reference to the problem of retrolental fibroplasia. Br J Ophthalmol. 1954;38(7):397–432. https://doi.org/10.1136/bjo.38.7.397.

Autrata R, Krejcírová I, Senková K, Holoušová M, Doležel Z, Borek I. Intravitreal pegaptanib combined with diode laser therapy for stage 3+ retinopathy of prematurity in zone I and posterior zone II. Eur J Ophthalmol. 2012;22(5):687–94. https://doi.org/10.5301/ejo.5000166.

Aydemir O, Sarikabadayi YU, Aydemir C, et al. Adjusted poor weight gain for birth weight and gestational age as a predictor of severe ROP in VLBW infants. Eye (Lond). 2011;25(6):725–9. https://doi.org/10.1038/eye.2011.29.

Binenbaum G, Bell EF, Donohue P, et al. Development of modified screening criteria for retinopathy of prematurity: primary results from the postnatal growth and retinopathy of prematurity study. JAMA Ophthalmol. 2018;136(9):1034–40. https://doi.org/10.1001/jamaophthalmol.2018.2753.

Cavallaro G, Filippi L, Bagnoli P, et al. The pathophysiology of retinopathy of prematurity: an update of previous and recent knowledge. Acta Ophthalmol. 2014;92(1):2–20. https://doi.org/10.1111/aos.12049.

Cayabyab R, Ramanathan R. Retinopathy of prematurity: therapeutic strategies based on pathophysiology. Neonatology. 2016;109(4):369–76. https://doi.org/10.1159/000444901.

Cerman E, Ozarslan Ozcan D, Celiker H, Eraslan M, Sahin O, Kazokoglu H. Late clinical characteristics of infants with retinopathy of prematurity and treated with cryotherapy. Int J Ophthalmol. 2016;9(4):567–71. https://doi.org/10.18240/ijo.2016.04.15.

Chan-Ling T, Gole GA, Quinn GE, Adamson SJ, Darlow BA. Pathophysiology, screening and treatment of ROP: a multi-disciplinary perspective. Prog Retin Eye Res. 2018;62:77–119. https://doi.org/10.1016/j.preteyeres.2017.09.002.

Chee RI, Darwish D, Fernandez-Vega A, et al. Retinal telemedicine. Curr Ophthalmol Rep. 2018;6(1):36–45. https://doi.org/10.1007/s40135-018-0161-8.

Chiang MF, Melia M, Buffenn AN, et al. Detection of clinically significant retinopathy of prematurity using wide-angle digital retinal photography: a report by the American Academy of Ophthalmology. Ophthalmology. 2012;119(6):1272–80. https://doi.org/10.1016/j.ophtha.2012.01.002.

Choi J, Kim JH, Kim SJ, Yu YS. Long-term results of lens-sparing vitrectomy for progressive posterior-type stage 4A retinopathy of prematurity. Korean J Ophthalmol. 2012;26(4):277–84. https://doi.org/10.3341/kjo.2012.26.4.277.

Connolly BP, Ng EY, McNamara JA, Regillo CD, Vander JF, Tasman W. A comparison of laser photocoagulation with cryotherapy for threshold retinopathy of prematurity at 10 years: Part 2. Refractive outcome. Ophthalmology. 2002;109(5):936–41. https://doi.org/10.1016/s0161-6420(01)01015-6.

Eckert GU, Fortes Filho JB, Maia M, Procianoy RS. A predictive score for retinopathy of prematurity in very low birth weight preterm infants. Eye (Lond). 2012;26(3):400–6. https://doi.org/10.1038/eye.2011.334.

Fijalkowski N, Zheng LL, Henderson MT, Wallenstein MB, Leng T, Moshfeghi DM. Stanford University Network for Diagnosis of Retinopathy of Prematurity (SUNDROP): four-years of screening with telemedicine. Curr Eye Res. 2013;38(2):283–91. https://doi.org/10.3109/02713683.2012.754902.

Flynn JT, Tasman W. Retinopathy of prematurity: a clinicians guide. Springer; 1992.

Fortes Filho JB, Bonomo PP, Maia M, Procianoy RS. Weight gain measured at 6 weeks after birth as a predictor for severe retinopathy of prematurity: study with 317 very low birth weight preterm babies. Graefes Arch Clin Exp Ophthalmol. 2009;247(6):831–6. https://doi.org/10.1007/s00417-008-1012-3.

Gilbert C. Retinopathy of prematurity: a global perspective of the epidemics, population of babies at risk and implications for control. Early Hum Dev. 2008;84(2):77–82. https://doi.org/10.1016/j.earlhumdev.2007.11.009.

Good WV, Group ETfRoPC. Final results of the Early Treatment for Retinopathy of Prematurity (ETROP) randomized trial. Trans Am Ophthalmol Soc. 2004;102:233–48; discussion 248-50.

Group CfRoPC. Multicenter Trial of Cryotherapy for Retinopathy of Prematurity: ophthalmological outcomes at 10 years. Arch Ophthalmol. 2001;119(8):1110–8. https://doi.org/10.1001/archopht.119.8.1110.

Gunay M, Sukgen EA, Celik G, Kocluk Y. Comparison of bevacizumab, ranibizumab, and laser photocoagulation in the treatment of retinopathy of prematurity in Turkey. Curr Eye Res. 2017;42(3):462–9. https://doi.org/10.1080/02713683.2016.1196709.

Gupta MP, Chan RVP, Anzures R, et al. Practice patterns in retinopathy of prematurity treatment for disease milder than recommended by guidelines. Am J Ophthalmol. 2016;163:1–10. https://doi.org/10.1016/j.ajo.2015.12.005.

Harder BC, Schlichtenbrede FC, von Baltz S, Jendritza W, Jendritza B, Jonas JB. Intravitreal bevacizumab for retinopathy of prematurity: refractive error results. Am J Ophthalmol. 2013;155(6):1119–1124.e1. https://doi.org/10.1016/j.ajo.2013.01.014.

Huang CY, Lien R, Wang NK, et al. Changes in systemic vascular endothelial growth factor levels after intravitreal injection of aflibercept in infants with retinopathy of prematurity. Graefes Arch Clin Exp Ophthalmol. 2018;256(3):479–87. https://doi.org/10.1007/s00417-017-3878-4.

Hwang CK, Hubbard GB, Hutchinson AK, Lambert SR. Outcomes after intravitreal bevacizumab versus laser photocoagulation for retinopathy of prematurity: a 5-year retrospective analysis. Ophthalmology. 2015;122(5):1008–15. https://doi.org/10.1016/j.ophtha.2014.12.017.

Isaac M, Mireskandari K, Tehrani N. Treatment of type 1 retinopathy of prematurity with bevacizumab versus laser. J AAPOS. 2015;19(2):140–4. https://doi.org/10.1016/j.jaapos.2015.01.009.

Jackson KM, Scott KE, Graff Zivin J, et al. Cost-utility analysis of telemedicine and ophthalmoscopy for retinopathy of prematurity management. Arch Ophthalmol. 2008;126(4):493–9. https://doi.org/10.1001/archopht.126.4.493.

Lien R, Yu MH, Hsu KH, et al. Neurodevelopmental outcomes in infants with retinopathy of prematurity and bevacizumab treatment. PLoS One. 2016;11(1):e0148019. https://doi.org/10.1371/journal.pone.0148019.

Löfqvist C, Hansen-Pupp I, Andersson E, et al. Validation of a new retinopathy of prematurity screening method monitoring longitudinal postnatal weight and insulinlike growth factor I. Arch Ophthalmol. 2009;127(5):622–7. https://doi.org/10.1001/archophthalmol.2009.69.

McNamara JA, Tasman W, Vander JF, Brown GC. Diode laser photocoagulation for retinopathy of prematurity. Preliminary results. Arch Ophthalmol. 1992;110(12):1714–6. https://doi.org/10.1001/archopht.1992.01080240054029.

Mintz-Hittner HA, Kennedy KA, Chuang AZ, Group B-RC. Efficacy of intravitreal bevacizumab for stage 3+ retinopathy of prematurity. N Engl J Med. 2011;364(7):603–15. https://doi.org/10.1056/NEJMoa1007374.

Mintz-Hittner HA, Geloneck MM, Chuang AZ. Clinical management of recurrent retinopathy of prematurity after intravitreal bevacizumab monotherapy. Ophthalmology. 2016;123(9):1845–55. https://doi.org/10.1016/j.ophtha.2016.04.028.

Morin J, Luu TM, Superstein R, et al. Neurodevelopmental outcomes following bevacizumab injections for retinopathy of prematurity. Pediatrics. 2016;137(4) https://doi.org/10.1542/peds.2015-3218.

Mueller B, Salchow DJ, Waffenschmidt E, et al. Treatment of type I ROP with intravitreal bevacizumab or laser photocoagulation according to retinal zone. Br J Ophthalmol. 2017;101(3):365–70. https://doi.org/10.1136/bjophthalmol-2016-308375.

Nagata M, Yamagishi N, Ikeda S. Summarized results of treatment of acute proliferative retinopathy of prematurity during the past 15 years in Tenri Hospital. Nippon Ganka Gakkai Zasshi. 1982;86(9):1236–44.

Pérez-Muñuzuri A, Fernández-Lorenzo JR, Couce-Pico ML, Blanco-Teijeiro MJ, Fraga-Bermúdez JM. Serum levels of IGF1 are a useful predictor of retinopathy of prematurity. Acta Paediatr. 2010;99(4):519–25. https://doi.org/10.1111/j.1651-2227.2009.01677.x.

Phelps DL. Retinopathy of prematurity. N Engl J Med. 1992;326(16):1078–80. https://doi.org/10.1056/NEJM199204163261609.

Pieh C, Krüger M, Lagrèze WA, et al. Plasma sE-selectin in premature infants: a possible surrogate marker of retinopathy of prematurity. Invest Ophthalmol Vis Sci. 2010;51(7):3709–13. https://doi.org/10.1167/iovs.09-4723.

Piyasena C, Dhaliwal C, Russell H, et al. Prediction of severe retinopathy of prematurity using the WINROP algorithm in a birth cohort in South East Scotland. Arch Dis Child Fetal Neonatal Ed. 2014;99(1):F29–33. https://doi.org/10.1136/archdischild-2013-304101.

Prematurity ICftCoRo. The International Classification of Retinopathy of Prematurity revisited. Arch Ophthalmol. 2005;123(7):991–9. https://doi.org/10.1001/archopht.123.7.991.

Quinn GE. Retinopathy of prematurity blindness worldwide: phenotypes in the third epidemic. Eye Brain. 2016;8:31–6. https://doi.org/10.2147/EB.S94436.

Rezai KA, Eliott D, Ferrone PJ, Kim RW. Near confluent laser photocoagulation for the treatment of threshold retinopathy of prematurity. Arch Ophthalmol. 2005;123(5):621–6. https://doi.org/10.1001/archopht.123.5.621.

Sankar MJ, Sankar J, Chandra P. Anti-vascular endothelial growth factor (VEGF) drugs for treatment of retinopathy of prematurity. Cochrane Database Syst Rev. 2018;(1):CD009734. https://doi.org/10.1002/14651858.CD009734.pub3.

Shah PK, Narendran V, Kalpana N, Gilbert C. Severe retinopathy of prematurity in big babies in India: history repeating itself? Indian J Pediatr. 2009;76(8):801–4. https://doi.org/10.1007/s12098-009-0175-1.

Shalev B, Farr AK, Repka MX. Randomized comparison of diode laser photocoagulation versus cryotherapy for threshold retinopathy of prematurity: seven-year outcome. Am J Ophthalmol. 2001;132(1):76–80. https://doi.org/10.1016/s0002-9394(01)00956-4.

Shapiro MJ, Alpert J, Pandit RT. Tent-shaped retinal detachments in retinopathy of prematurity. Retina. 2006;26(7 Suppl):S32–7. https://doi.org/10.1097/01.iae.0000244284.79004.af.

Silva RA, Murakami Y, Lad EM, Moshfeghi DM. Stanford University network for diagnosis of retinopathy of prematurity (SUNDROP): 36-month experience with telemedicine screening. Ophthalmic Surg Lasers Imaging. 2011;42(1):12–9. https://doi.org/10.3928/15428877-20100929-08.

Smith LE. Pathogenesis of retinopathy of prematurity. Growth Horm IGF Res. 2004;14 Suppl A:S140–4. https://doi.org/10.1016/j.ghir.2004.03.030.

Spiegel PH, Lisa S. Thomson. Handbook of pediatric retinal disease: Springer; 2006.

Stone J, Itin A, Alon T, et al. Development of retinal vasculature is mediated by hypoxia-induced vascular endothelial growth factor (VEGF) expression by neuroglia. J Neurosci. 1995;15(7 Pt 1):4738–47.

Terry TL. Fibroblastic overgrowth of persistent tunica vasculosa lentis in infants born prematurely: II. Report of cases-clinical aspects. Trans Am Ophthalmol Soc. 1942;40:262–84.

VanderVeen DK, Cataltepe SU. Anti-vascular endothelial growth factor intravitreal therapy for retinopathy of prematurity. Semin Perinatol. 2019;43(6):375–80. https://doi.org/10.1053/j.semperi.2019.05.011.

Wallace DK, Freedman SF, Hartnett ME, Quinn GE. Predictive value of pre-plus disease in retinopathy of prematurity. Arch Ophthalmol. 2011;129(5):591–6. https://doi.org/10.1001/archophthalmol.2011.63.

Wallace DK, Kraker RT, Freedman SF, et al. Assessment of lower doses of intravitreous bevacizumab for retinopathy of prematurity: a phase 1 dosing study. JAMA Ophthalmol. 2017;135(6):654–6. https://doi.org/10.1001/jamaophthalmol.2017.1055.

Wu AL, Wu WC. Anti-VEGF for ROP and pediatric retinal diseases. Asia Pac J Ophthalmol (Phila). 2018;7(3):145–51. https://doi.org/10.22608/APO.201837.

Wu WC, Lien R, Liao PJ, et al. Serum levels of vascular endothelial growth factor and related factors after intravitreous bevacizumab injection for retinopathy of prematurity. JAMA Ophthalmol. 2015;133(4):391–7. https://doi.org/10.1001/jamaophthalmol.2014.5373.

Wu WC, Shih CP, Lien R, et al. SERUM VASCULAR ENDOTHELIAL GROWTH FACTOR AFTER BEVACIZUMAB OR RANIBIZUMAB TREATMENT FOR RETINOPATHY OF PREMATURITY. Retina. 2017;37(4):694–701. https://doi.org/10.1097/IAE.0000000000001209.

Zepeda-Romero LC, Hård AL, Gomez-Ruiz LM, et al. Prediction of retinopathy of prematurity using the screening algorithm WINROP in a Mexican population of preterm infants. Arch Ophthalmol. 2012;130(6):720–3. https://doi.org/10.1001/archophthalmol.2012.215.

Zhang G, Yang M, Zeng J, et al. COMPARISON OF INTRAVITREAL INJECTION OF RANIBIZUMAB VERSUS LASER THERAPY FOR ZONE II TREATMENT-REQUIRING RETINOPATHY OF PREMATURITY. Retina. 2017;37(4):710–7. https://doi.org/10.1097/IAE.0000000000001241.

Anti-VEGF for Retinopathy of Prematurity

3

An-Lun Wu and Wei-Chi Wu

Introduction

Retinopathy of prematurity (ROP) is one of the major vasoproliferative disorders of the retina that is associated with severe visual impairment in premature infants. Because vascular endothelial growth factor (VEGF) plays a key role in the pathogenesis of ROP, the use of anti-VEGF agents has been found to be an effective treatment for ROP (Fig. 3.1), has gradually gained popularity, and has even been advocated as first-line therapy by some ophthalmologists (Chen et al. 2015; Hwang et al. 2015; Mintz-Hittner et al. 2011; Sankar et al. 2016).

Ablation of the avascular retina by either cryotherapy or laser photocoagulation, as shown in the Cryotherapy for Retinopathy of Prematurity study (CRYO-ROP) (Cryotherapy for Retinopathy of Prematurity Cooperative Group 1988) and the Early Treatment for Retinopathy of Prematurity (ETROP) study (Early Treatment For Retinopathy Of Prematurity Cooperative 2003), has been a useful and effective treatment for ROP; however, there are several potential advantages of anti-VEGF treatment over these conventional forms of management (Mintz-Hittner 2012; Klufas and Chan 2015). First, anti-VEGF injection may allow normal vasculature to further vascularize toward the peripheral retina (Fig. 3.2), reducing the possible permanent visual field defect. Secondly, the administration of anti-VEGF is a short procedure and therefore can be done at the bedside under sedation only. On the contrary, laser photocoagulation often needs to be performed with intubation and sedation, or under general anesthesia, because it is a time-consuming procedure. Third, anti-VEGF agents are able to neutralize the VEGF in the vitreous fluid directly, but the peripheral retina ablative procedure destroys the peripheral retina and inhibits the production of VEGF. Thus, laser photocoagulation does not affect the VEGF already present in the vitreous fluid, but anti-VEGF agents are able to inactivate VEGF directly, and may have a more rapid response than laser photocoagulation. Further, it has been suggested that ROP treated with anti-VEGF is more likely to remain emmetropic and less likely to develop myopia or high myopia as compared with laser treatment (Chen et al. 2014; Geloneck et al. 2014). Finally, intravitreal injection of anti-VEGF may still be given in cases with hazy media, including cornea or lens vitreous opacity, presence of tunica vasculosa lentis, and poor pupillary dilation. It would be difficult to apply laser photocoagulation in patients with hazy media and poor visualization of the retina.

However, some uncertainties remain regarding the use of anti-VEGF in the treatment of ROP, such as the appropriate dose of anti-VEGF agents in newborns; follow-up frequency; the fate of peripheral avascular retina; long-term effects of anti-VEGF therapy on visual acuity and visual fields; and whether there are neurodevelopmental defects after systemic VEGF suppression following the use of anti-VEGF agents.

ROP Pathogenesis and Clinical Studies

The pathogenesis of ROP involves two discrete phases. Phase I occurs from roughly 22 to 30 weeks' postmenstrual age, and involves relative hyperoxia and decreased VEGF levels. Phase II occurs from roughly 31 to 44 weeks' postmenstrual age; it is now understood that this period is at high risk for ROP development, because hypoxia of phase II can induce a rapid increase in VEGF-promoting neovascularization (Smith 2008; Mintz-Hittner et al. 2011). Consequently, injection of anti-VEGF therapy with appropriate timing—when VEGF in the ROP eyes is highly expressed—is crucially important. It not only acts against the already released VEGF, but also prevents the release of further VEGF if the normal vasculature continues toward the peripheral retina.

Recently multiple studies have demonstrated the efficacy of intravitreal anti-VEGF therapy in promoting regression of ROP. A prospective randomized multicenter trial by the

A.-L. Wu · W.-C. Wu (✉)
Department of Ophthalmology, Chang-Gung Memorial Hospital, Linkou, Taoyuan, Taiwan

R. V. P. Chan (ed.), *Pediatric Retinal Diseases*, Retina Atlas, https://doi.org/10.1007/978-981-19-1364-8_3

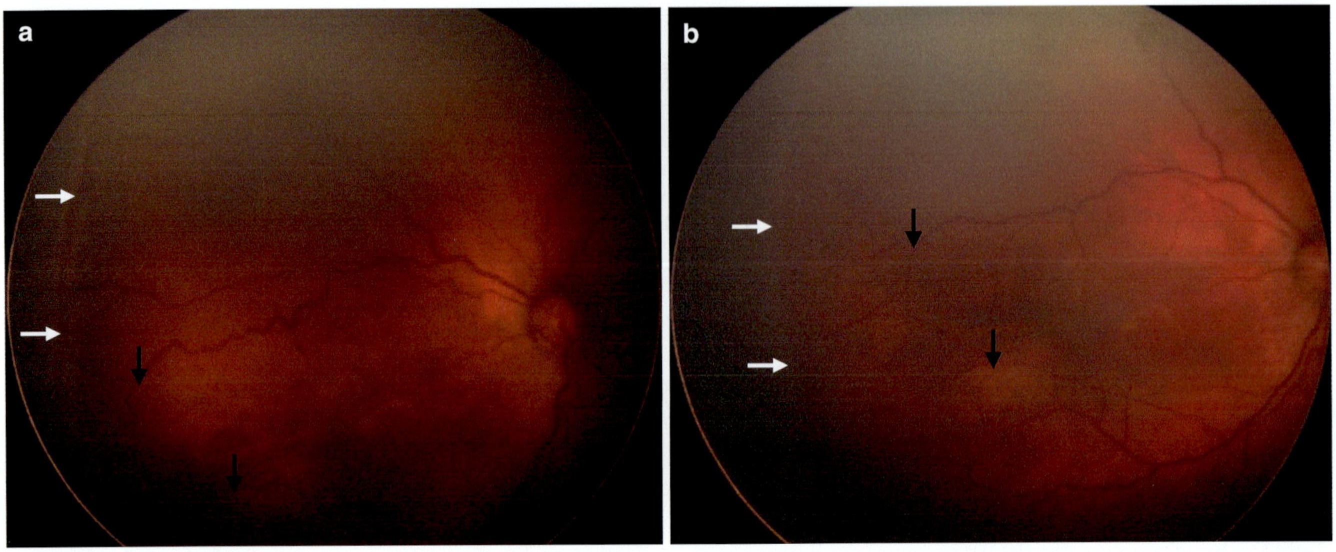

Fig. 3.1 Fundus photographs showing stage 3 retinopathy of prematurity, before and after bevacizumab treatment. (**a**) Before the injection of bevacizumab, neovascularization is seen with avascular retina in the periphery. (**b**) After injection of bevacizumab, neovascularization has regressed and retinal vascularization has continued toward the retinal periphery. White arrows indicate the extent of vascularization; black arrows indicate identical retinal points for comparison before and after treatment

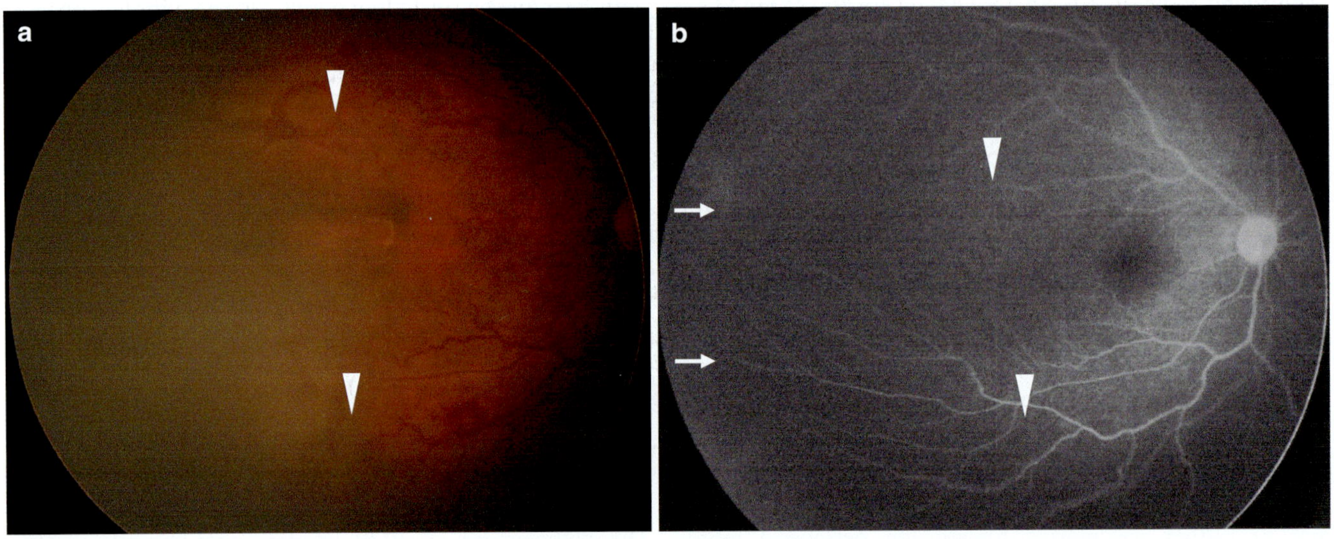

Fig. 3.2 Fundus photograph and fluorescein angiogram of an infant with zone I, stage 3 retinopathy of prematurity, before and after anti-VEGF treatment. (**a**) Before injection of bevacizumab, prominent plus disease with flat neovascularization in zone 1 was demonstrated in a case of aggressive posterior retinopathy of prematurity (APROP). (**b**) After the injection of bevacizumab at 18 months' postmenstrual age, fluorescein angiogram showed continued vascularization of the peripheral retina in zone III. Arrowheads indicate the extent of vascularization in zone I at the time of treatment with bevacizumab, and arrows indicate the extent of vascularization after treatment

Bevacizumab Eliminates the Angiogenic Threat of Retinopathy of Prematurity (BEAT-ROP) Cooperative Group assessed the efficacy of bevacizumab monotherapy in the treatment of premature patients with ROP in zone I or posterior zone II, as compared with conventional laser therapy (Mintz-Hittner et al. 2011). The study concluded that intravitreal bevacizumab monotherapy showed a significant treatment benefit with bevacizumab over laser for zone I, stage 3 plus ROP.

Our group has conducted multicenter studies in Taiwan using intravitreal injection of bevacizumab (IVB) to treat high-risk prethreshold ROP (*type 1* ROP), and these studies have showed promising outcomes in the Asian population (Wu et al. 2013). Tunica vasculosa lentis (Fig. 3.3) and plus disease (Fig. 3.4) both respond quickly to anti-VEGF treatment. Nevertheless, it is very important to follow up with the patient, because treatment with anti-VEGF is not a once-and-done therapy (Moshfeghi and Berrocal 2011). Infants treated

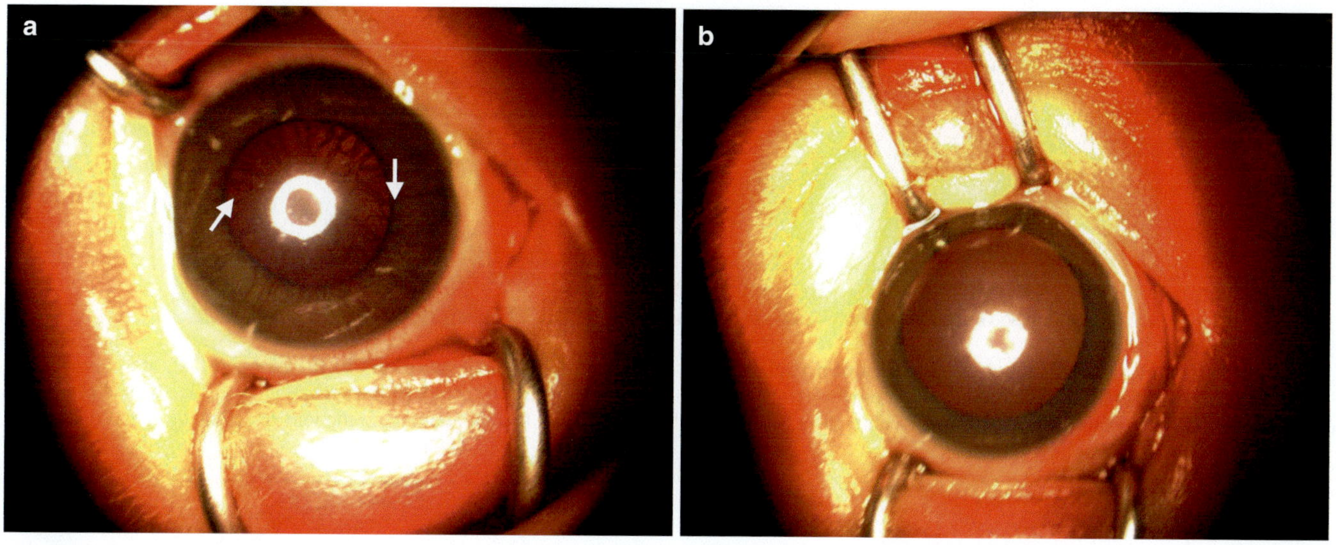

Fig. 3.3 Regression of tunica vasculosa lentis in the right eye of a patient with stage 3 ROP after injection of aflibercept. (**a**) Prominent tunica vasculosa lentis is noted, and the pupil was not well dilated before injection of aflibercept (arrows). (**b**) One week later, after aflibercept injection, the pupil is fully dilated, and the tunica vasculosalentis has disappeared

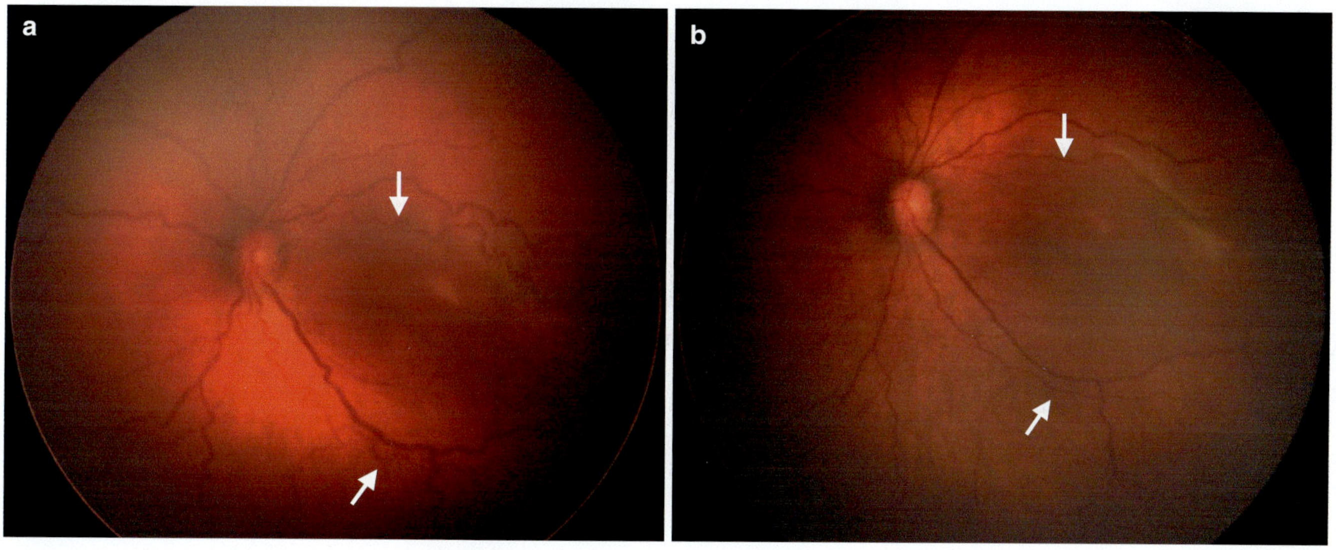

Fig. 3.4 Regression of plus disease in the left eye of a patient with stage 3 ROP, following injection of bevacizumab. (**a**) Fundus photography shows the tortuosity and dilatation of retinal vessels (arrows) in this ROP patient, prior to treatment. (**b**) One week later, after bevacizumab injection, the tortuosity and dilatation of retinal vessels have decreased (arrows)

with anti-VEGF should be carefully watched in a prolonged follow-up because of possible late recurrence (Hu et al. 2012).

Injection Technique

The injection technique in pediatric eyes is different from that used in adult eyes. Surgeons need to be very familiar with the technique before applying this treatment, in order to avoid damaging either the lens or the retina, because the lens is larger relative to the overall ocular volume in newborns' eyes. There are certain considerations for the intravitreal injection technique in newborns, including the appropriate injection site, needle gauge, and injection angle (Wu et al. 2013). After aseptic procedures, the injection should be performed with a 30-gauge needle at the pars plicata (Fig. 3.5), because the pars plana is not fully developed in newborns. Furthermore, the injection angle begins almost perpendicular to the globe, but is then slightly directed toward the center of the eyeball, after the needle has passed the lens equator (Fig. 3.6). Potential complications associated with intravitreal injection, including cataract, endophthalmitis, and retinal detachment, need to be monitored for closely after anti-VEGF injection.

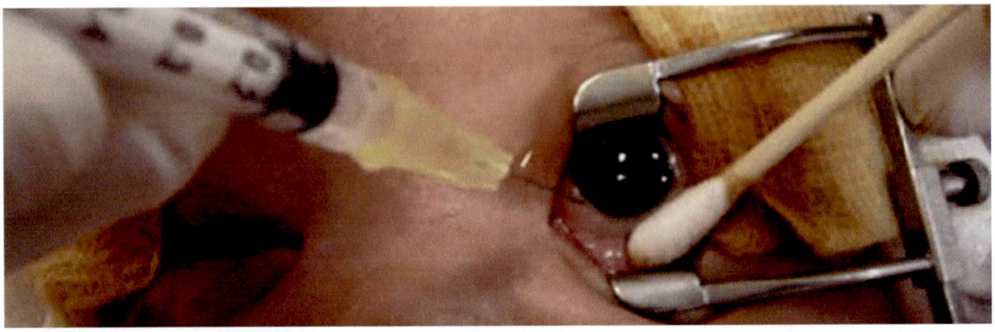

Fig. 3.5 Photograph showing intravitreal injection of bevacizumab at the pars plicata for a patient with retinopathy of prematurity. After aseptic procedures, the injection was performed with a 30-gauge needle directed almost perpendicularly to the globe at first, and then slightly directed toward the center of the eyeball after the needle had passed the lens equator, to avoid damaging the lens or retina

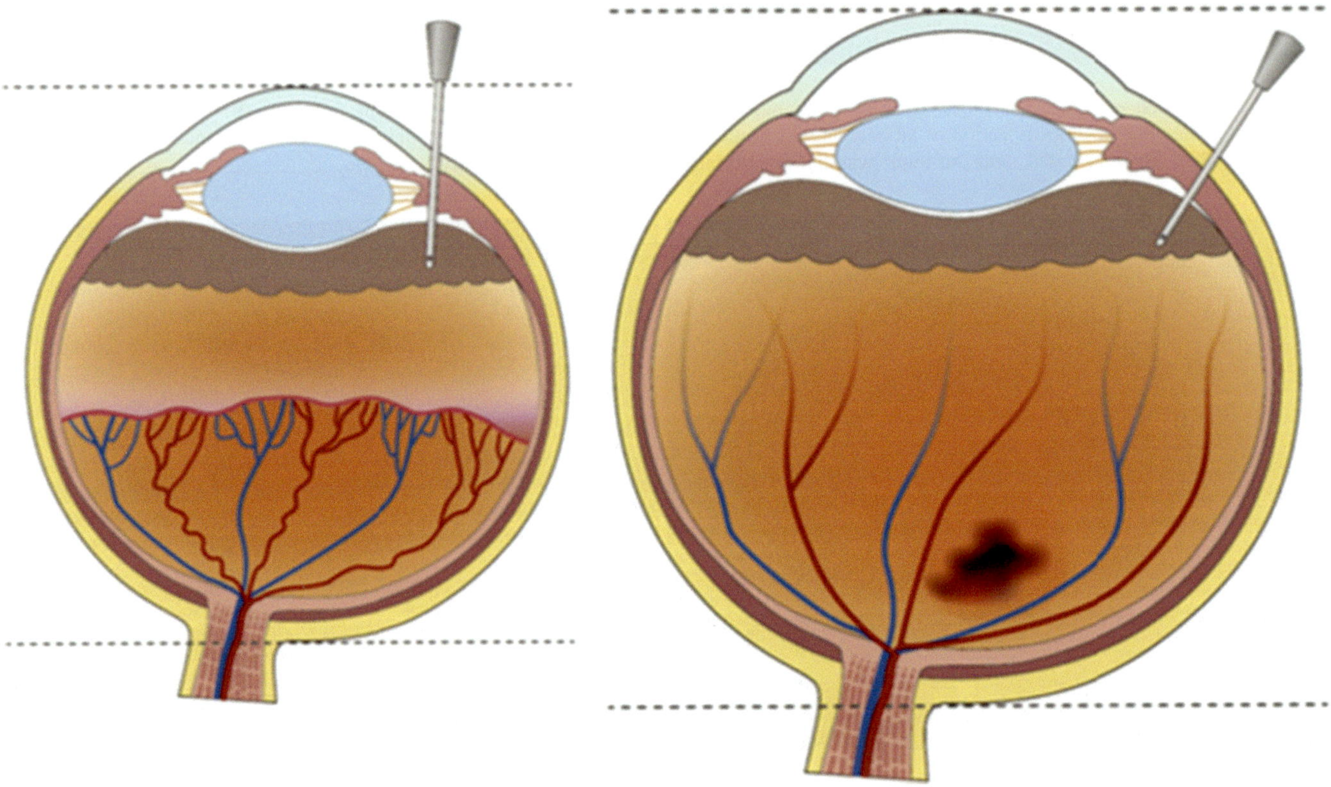

Fig. 3.6 Diagrams showing a comparison of the intravitreal injection angle in newborns (left) and adults (right). (Left) For the intravitreal injection of bevacizumab in newborn patients with retinopathy of prematurity, the injection is performed at the pars plicata, because the pars plana is not fully developed in newborns. Therefore, the injection angle is almost perpendicular to the globe. (Right) For the intravitreal injection of bevacizumab in adult patients with age-related macular degeneration, the injection is performed at the pars plana, and the injection angle is directed toward the center of the globe

Different Types of Anti-VEGF and Treatment Dose

Anti-VEGF agents for ROP include bevacizumab (Avastin; Genentech Inc., South San Francisco, CA, USA), ranibizumab (Lucentis; Genentech Inc., South San Francisco, CA, USA), pegaptanib (Macugen; Eyetech Inc., Cedar Knolls, NJ, USA), and aflibercept (Eylea; Regeneron Pharmaceuticals, Tarrytown, NY, USA). Each of them has different pharmacokinetic effects, molecular sizes, structures, and half-lives (Autrata et al. 2012; Chen et al. 2015; Geloneck et al. 2014; Gunay et al. 2017; Hwang et al. 2015; Lee et al. 2010; Lepore et al. 2014; Moran et al. 2014; Zhang et al. 2017; Mintz-Hittner et al. 2011). Bevacizumab and ranibizumab are the more commonly used agents for treating ROP. Bevacizumab is a full monoclonal antibody and was the first anti-VEGF used for the treatment of ROP. A much

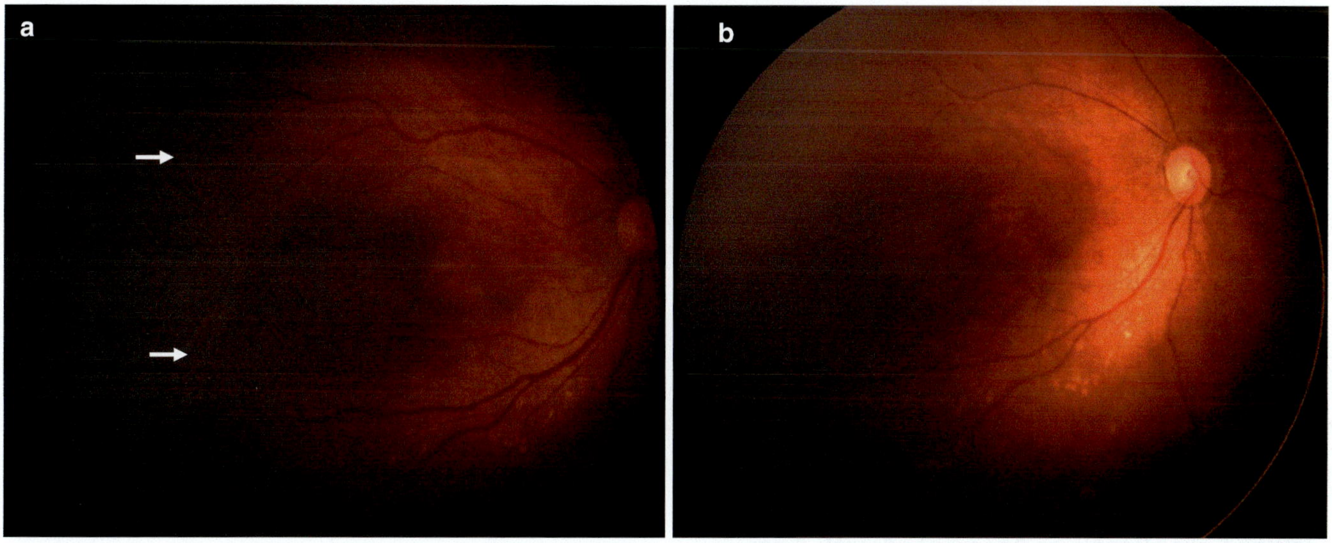

Fig. 3.7 Fundus photographs showing regression of stage 3 retinopathy of prematurity following ranibizumab treatment. (**a**) Before the injection of ranibizumab, neovascularization (arrows) is seen with avascular retina in the periphery. (**b**) After treatment, fundus photography shows gradual regression of extraretinal neovascularization, and continued vascularization of the peripheral retina

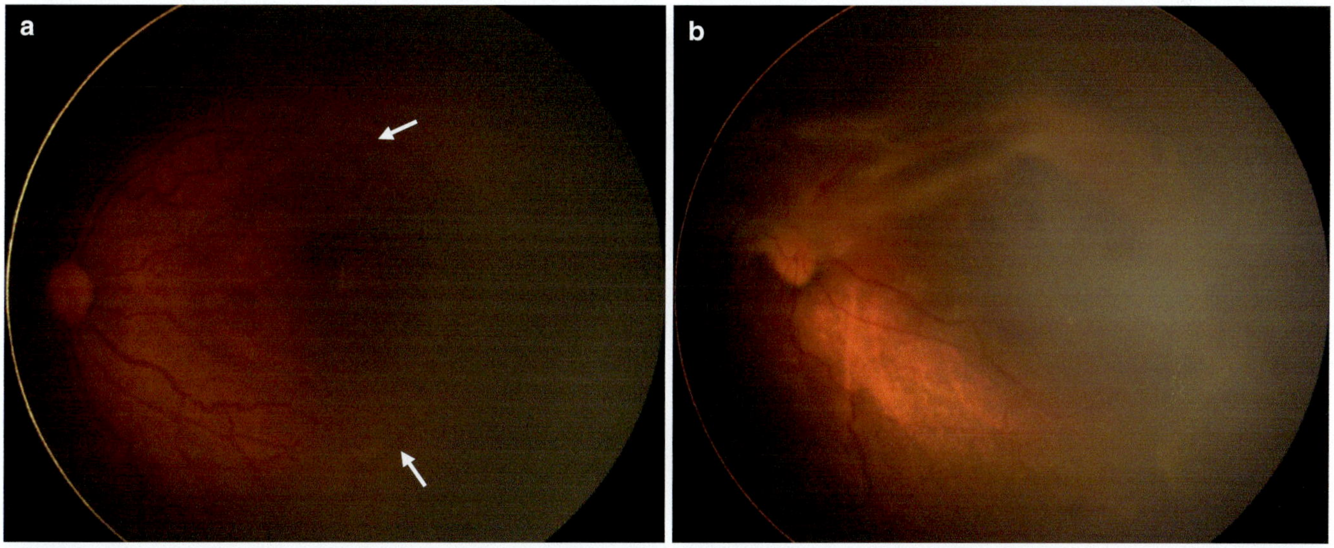

Fig. 3.8 Fundus photographs from a male infant with anemia and bronchopulmonary dysplasia, weighing 1820 g and at 31 weeks of gestation at birth, demonstrate aggressive posterior retinopathy of prematurity (APROP) in zone 1 that did not respond to bevacizumab injection. (**a**) Fundus photography prior to bevacizumab treatment demonstrates plus disease and flat new vessels (arrows) in zone 1. (**b**) After intravitreal injection of bevacizumab, extraretinal neovascularization and plus disease have persisted, and there is increased traction of the fibrovascular tissues, causing detached retina with macular involvement

smaller humanized monoclonal antibody Fab fragment, ranibizumab, was later used with the aim of being a safer treatment option (Fig. 3.7). Both bevacizumab and ranibizumab bind to all VEGF-A isoforms and have demonstrated efficacy in the treatment of Type 1 ROP; however, the rate of ROP recurrence (Fig. 3.8) has varied somewhat between different studies (Chen et al. 2015; Gunay et al. 2017).

One study has reported a higher rate of recurrence in ROP eyes treated with ranibizumab as compared with bevacizumab (Gunay et al. 2017). Our group performed a comparative case series study, using both bevacizumab and ranibizumab as the primary treatment for Type 1 ROP. Our results showed similar efficacy in disease regression and recurrence between these two drugs (Chen et al. 2015). There were no significant differences in mean refractive errors at 1 year of corrected age, though there was a higher chance of developing high myopia in the bevacizumab treatment group. However, other studies have suggested that ranibizumab-treated eyes have higher chances of recurrence, requiring further treatment (Chuluunbat et al. 2016).

There is no definite conclusion regarding what dose of any of the anti-VEGF medications is optimal for ROP (Harder et al. 2014; Lorenz et al. 2017). Most previous studies have used 0.625 mg/0.025 ml for bevacizumab and 0.25 mg/0.025 ml for ranibizumab, or half of the adult doses, per eye when applied. All of these anti-VEGF agents leak into systemic circulation after intravitreal injection, and that causes the suppression of systemic VEGF. We still do not know the long-term effects of suppressed VEGF after anti-VEGF use in these premature patients. Consequently, further investigation is warranted to provide guidance for dose selection.

Ocular Complications Associated with Anti-VEGF Agents

Although localized ocular complication rates in the literature have been low (Pertl et al. 2015), infants should be monitored for potential complications after intravitreal injection of anti-VEGF. Possible complications include cataracts, endophthalmitis, vitreous hemorrhage (Fig. 3.9), pre-retinal hemorrhage (Fig. 3.10), and retinal detachment.

In a multicenter study in Taiwan, we reported vitreous or pre-retinal hemorrhage in 8% of eyes and transient venous sheathing in 4% of eyes as complications of intravitreal bevacizumab injection; however, vitreous or pre-retinal hemorrhage had later resolved in all eyes, and sheathed vessels had reperfused at subsequent follow-up (Wu et al. 2011). Serious adverse events of retinal breaks and bilateral vascular attenuation with subretinal perivascular exudates and optic atrophy also occurred after IVB in a series report from India (Jalali et al. 2013).

Another concern from treatment-induced complication is termed "ROP crunch," which can occur quickly if anti-VEGF injection was performed when there was already significant traction on the retina (Fig. 3.11). This can accelerate membrane contraction and cause a significant increase of tractional retinal detachment, resulting in poor outcomes.

Systemic Safety Concerns

Intravitreal injection of anti-VEGF for ROP has been shown to be effective in treating ROP; however, systemic VEGF suppression after intravitreal injection of anti-VEGFs in newborns is a concern. Sato et al. have found evidence of systemic bevacizumab exposure after IVB (Sato et al. 2012). A study of ours has further shown that VEGF levels were depressed for 2 months after IVB in patients with type 1 ROP, due to the leakage of bevacizumab into systemic circulation (Wu et al. 2015). Recently, we conducted a prospective study to measure serum VEGF changes in patients treated with bevacizumab or ranibizumab. In comparison with bevacizumab, ranibizumab injection for ROP resulted in no or barely detected suppression of systemic VEGF (Wu et al. 2017).

A retrospective observational study has revealed that preterm infants treated with bevacizumab were at increased risk (as compared to laser) of severe neurodevelopmental dis-

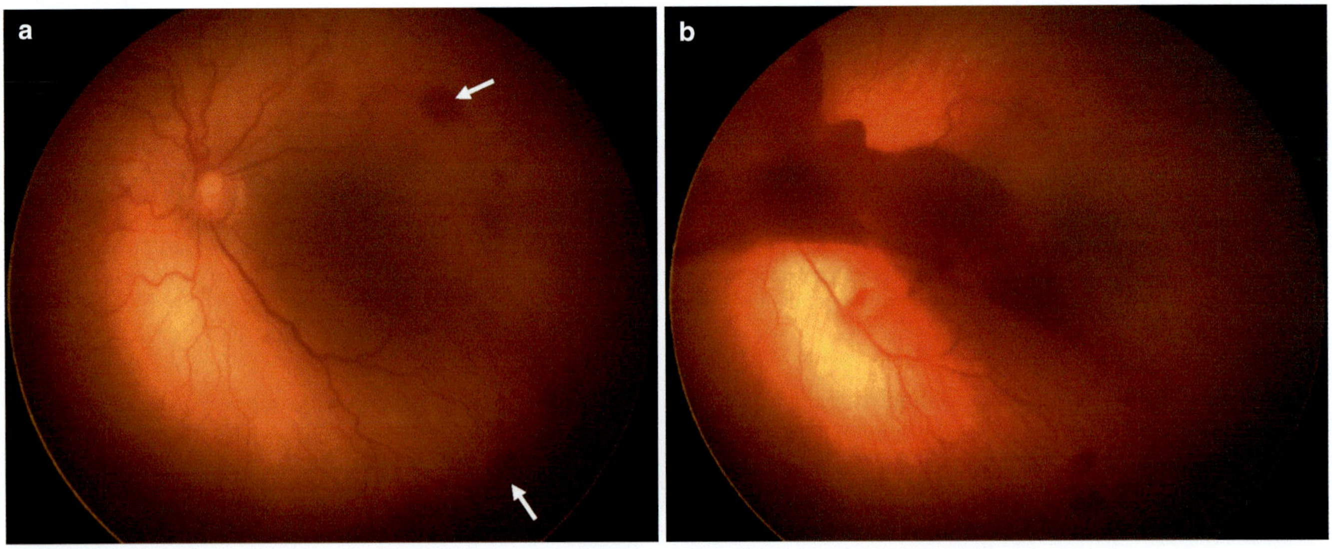

Fig. 3.9 Complication of vitreous hemorrhage after injection of aflibercept in the left eye of a patient with aggressive posterior retinopathy of prematurity (APROP). (**a**) Fundus photograph prior to aflibercept injection demonstrates zone I ROP with plus disease, flat neovascularization, and some pre-retinal hemorrhages (arrows) that were consistent with the characteristics of APROP. (**b**) After injection of aflibercept, the retinal vessel tortuosity has decreased, but vitreous hemorrhage is present

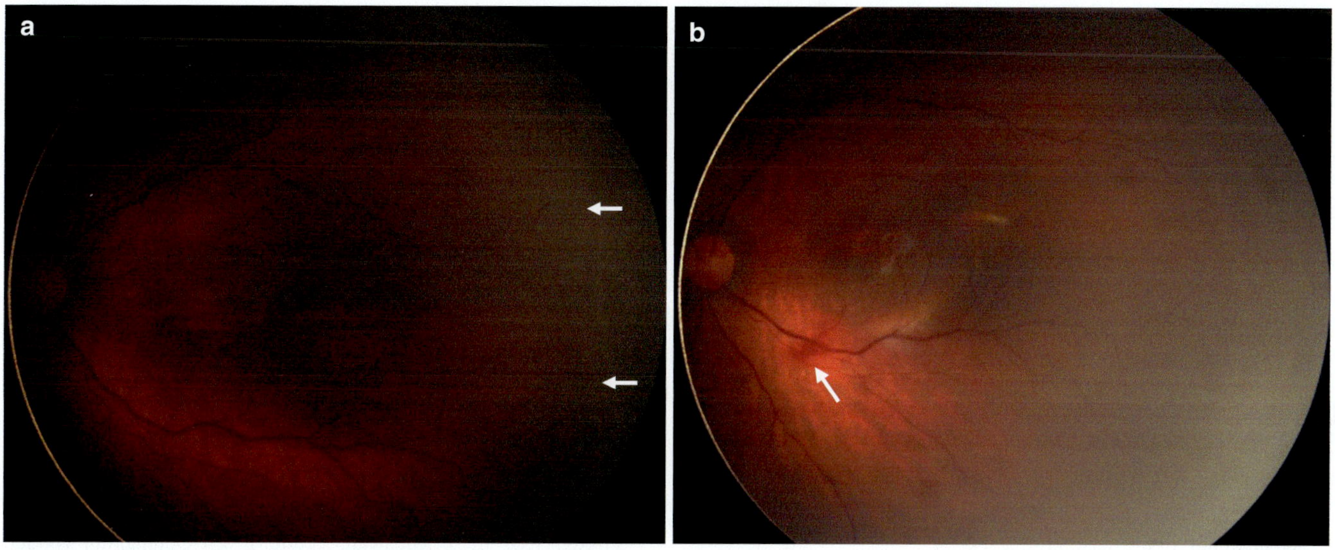

Fig. 3.10 Complications of pre-retinal hemorrhage following bevacizumab injection for retinopathy of prematurity. (**a**) Before the injection of bevacizumab, stage 3 retinopathy of prematurity with neovascularization (arrows) is seen in the peripheral retina. (**b**) After the bevacizumab injection, fundus photography shows gradual regression of extraretinal neovascularization and continued vascularization of the peripheral retina, but pre-retinal hemorrhage is observed

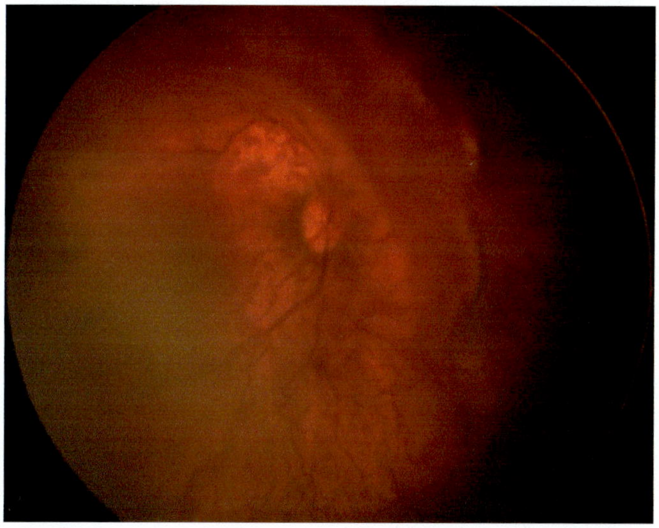

Fig. 3.11 Fibrotic traction and retinal detachment increase rapidly over the nasal area in the right eye in a stage 4A ROP patient, following injection of bevacizumab

abilities (Morin et al. 2016). However, several limitations, including the retrospective nature of the study, selection bias, and confounding factors, render its conclusions uncertain. In contrast, our group did not find worse neurodevelopmental outcomes in infants who received only bevacizumab, as compared to those treated with laser photocoagulation. But infants who required rescue therapy with laser or bevacizumab injection after initial, unsuccessful treatment, and patients with more severe disease status (i.e., in the end, both laser + IVB were given), showed some detrimental, neurodevelopmental effects (Lien et al. 2016). Questions remain about late systemic and neurodevelopmental effects after anti-VEGF therapy for ROP patients, so more data is needed in the future to objectively assess the effects of anti-VEGF in premature babies.

References

Autrata R, Krejcirova I, Senkova K, et al. Intravitreal pegaptanib combined with diode laser therapy for stage 3+ retinopathy of prematurity in zone I and posterior zone II. Eur J Ophthalmol. 2012;22:687–94.

Chen YH, Chen SN, Lien RI, et al. Refractive errors after the use of bevacizumab for the treatment of retinopathy of prematurity: 2-year outcomes. Eye (Lond). 2014;28:1080–6; quiz 1087.

Chen SN, Lian I, Hwang YC, et al. Intravitreal anti-vascular endothelial growth factor treatment for retinopathy of prematurity: comparison between Ranibizumab and Bevacizumab. Retina. 2015;35:667–74.

Chuluunbat T, Chan RV, Wang NK, et al. Nonresponse and recurrence of retinopathy of prematurity after intravitreal ranibizumab treatment. Ophthalmic Surg Lasers Imaging Retina. 2016;47:1095–105.

Cryotherapy for Retinopathy of Prematurity Cooperative Group. Multicenter trial of cryotherapy for retinopathy of prematurity. Preliminary results. Arch Ophthalmol. 1988;106:471–9.

Early Treatment For Retinopathy Of Prematurity Cooperative G. Revised indications for the treatment of retinopathy of prematurity: results of the early treatment for retinopathy of prematurity randomized trial. Arch Ophthalmol. 2003;121:1684–94.

Geloneck MM, Chuang AZ, Clark WL, et al. Refractive outcomes following bevacizumab monotherapy compared with conventional laser treatment: a randomized clinical trial. JAMA Ophthalmol. 2014;132:1327–33.

Gunay M, Sukgen EA, Celik G, et al. Comparison of bevacizumab, ranibizumab, and laser photocoagulation in the treatment of retinopathy of prematurity in Turkey. Curr Eye Res. 2017;42:462–9.

Harder BC, von Baltz S, Jonas JB, et al. Intravitreal low-dosage bevacizumab for retinopathy of prematurity. Acta Ophthalmol. 2014;92:577–81.

Hu J, Blair MP, Shapiro MJ, et al. Reactivation of retinopathy of prematurity after bevacizumab injection. Arch Ophthalmol. 2012;130:1000–6.

Hwang CK, Hubbard GB, Hutchinson AK, et al. Outcomes after intravitreal bevacizumab versus laser photocoagulation for retinopathy of prematurity: a 5-year retrospective analysis. Ophthalmology. 2015;122:1008–15.

Jalali S, Balakrishnan D, Zeynalova Z, et al. Serious adverse events and visual outcomes of rescue therapy using adjunct bevacizumab to laser and surgery for retinopathy of prematurity. The Indian Twin Cities Retinopathy of Prematurity Screening database Report number 5. Arch Dis Child Fetal Neonatal Ed. 2013;98:F327–33.

Klufas MA, Chan RV. Intravitreal anti-VEGF therapy as a treatment for retinopathy of prematurity: what we know after 7 years. J Pediatr Ophthalmol Strabismus. 2015;52:77–84.

Lee JY, Chae JB, Yang SJ, et al. Effects of intravitreal bevacizumab and laser in retinopathy of prematurity therapy on the development of peripheral retinal vessels. Graefes Arch Clin Exp Ophthalmol. 2010;248:1257–62.

Lepore D, Quinn GE, Molle F, et al. Intravitreal bevacizumab versus laser treatment in type 1 retinopathy of prematurity: report on fluorescein angiographic findings. Ophthalmology. 2014;121:2212–9.

Lien R, Yu MH, Hsu KH, et al. Neurodevelopmental outcomes in infants with retinopathy of prematurity and bevacizumab treatment. PLoS One. 2016;11:e0148019.

Lorenz B, Stieger K, Jager M, et al. RETINAL VASCULAR DEVELOPMENT WITH 0.312 MG INTRAVITREAL BEVACIZUMAB TO TREAT SEVERE POSTERIOR RETINOPATHY OF PREMATURITY: a longitudinal fluorescein angiographic study. Retina. 2017;37:97–111.

Mintz-Hittner HA. Treatment of retinopathy of prematurity with vascular endothelial growth factor inhibitors. Early Hum Dev. 2012;88:937–41.

Mintz-Hittner HA, Kennedy KA, Chuang AZ, et al. Efficacy of intravitreal bevacizumab for stage 3+ retinopathy of prematurity. N Engl J Med. 2011;364:603–15.

Moran S, O'Keefe M, Hartnett C, et al. Bevacizumab versus diode laser in stage 3 posterior retinopathy of prematurity. Acta Ophthalmol. 2014;92:e496–7.

Morin J, Luu TM, Superstein R, et al. Neurodevelopmental outcomes following bevacizumab injections for retinopathy of prematurity. Pediatrics. 2016;137

Moshfeghi DM, Berrocal AM. Retinopathy of prematurity in the time of bevacizumab: incorporating the BEAT-ROP results into clinical practice. Ophthalmology. 2011;118:1227–8.

Pertl L, Steinwender G, Mayer C, et al. A systematic review and meta-analysis on the safety of vascular endothelial growth factor (VEGF) inhibitors for the treatment of retinopathy of prematurity. PLoS One. 2015;10:e0129383.

Sankar MJ, Sankar J, Mehta M, et al. Anti-vascular endothelial growth factor (VEGF) drugs for treatment of retinopathy of prematurity. Cochrane Database Syst Rev. 2016;2:CD009734.

Sato T, Wada K, Arahori H, et al. Serum concentrations of bevacizumab (avastin) and vascular endothelial growth factor in infants with retinopathy of prematurity. Am J Ophthalmol. 2012;153:327–333 e321.

Smith LE. Through the eyes of a child: understanding retinopathy through ROP the Friedenwald lecture. Invest Ophthalmol Vis Sci. 2008;49:5177–82.

Wu WC, Yeh PT, Chen SN, et al. Effects and complications of bevacizumab use in patients with retinopathy of prematurity: a multicenter study in taiwan. Ophthalmology. 2011;118:176–83.

Wu WC, Kuo HK, Yeh PT, et al. An updated study of the use of bevacizumab in the treatment of patients with prethreshold retinopathy of prematurity in taiwan. Am J Ophthalmol. 2013;155:150–158 e151.

Wu WC, Lien R, Liao PJ, et al. Serum levels of vascular endothelial growth factor and related factors after intravitreous bevacizumab injection for retinopathy of prematurity. JAMA Ophthalmol. 2015;133:391–7.

Wu WC, Shih CP, Lien R, et al. Serum vascular endothelial growth factor after bevacizumab or ranibizumab treatment for retinopathy of prematurity. Retina. 2017;37:694–701.

Zhang G, Yang M, Zeng J, et al. Comparison of intravitreal injection of ranibizumab versus laser therapy for Zone II treatment-requiring retinopathy of prematurity. Retina. 2017;37:710–7.

Surgical Management of Retinopathy of Prematurity

4

Irina De la Huerta and Antonio Capone Jr

Introduction

Untreated threshold retinopathy of prematurity leads to retinal detachment in over 40% of cases (Cryotherapy for Retinopathy of Prematurity Cooperative Group 1988, 1994). Peripheral retinal ablation is effective in preventing the progression to retinal detachment in the majority of eyes with ROP (Cryotherapy for Retinopathy of Prematurity Cooperative Group 1988, 1994; Good and Early Treatment for Retinopathy of Prematurity Cooperative Group 2004; Early Treatment for Retinopathy of Prematurity Cooperative Group 2003). In the Early Treatment for Retinopathy of Prematurity (ETROP) trial 9.1% of laser-treated eyes progressed to retinal detachment, however, the trial used a pattern of laser burns up to one spot diameter apart (Good and Early Treatment for Retinopathy of Prematurity Cooperative Group 2004; Early Treatment for Retinopathy of Prematurity Cooperative Group 2003). Studies using a denser, near-confluent, laser pattern have generally reported lower progression rates of 3–4% (Banach et al. 2000; Rezai et al. 2005). Conversely, detachments after laser treatment are more often seen in eyes with incomplete peripheral ablation, and in those with Aggressive Posterior ROP (APROP) in zone I or posterior zone II (Drenser et al. 2010; Gunn et al. 2014). Almost all eyes that progress after photoablation do so within 9 weeks of treatment and this well-described and predictable pattern facilitates early diagnosis and intervention.

In recent years the off-label use of anti-VEGF therapy for ROP has increased, driven by the ability to perform the procedure without general anesthesia, faster regression of neovascularization, and potential for continued retinal vascular development. However, treatment with anti-VEGF agents has been shown to upregulate the activity of profibrotic cytokines, and the resulting profibrotic state may drive progression to tractional retinal detachments (Yonekawa et al. 2017a; Sato et al. 2009; Funk et al. 2009). Progressive detachment after anti-VEGF therapy generally occurs within 3 months of the initial treatment but can occur as late as 2.5 years after the anti-VEGF administration (Snyder et al. 2016). The rates of progression to retinal detachment are not clearly known, due to the lack of long-term follow-up studies and relatively small sample sizes.

Once considered inoperable, retinal detachments in ROP have become amenable to surgical management through advancements in pathophysiologic knowledge and surgical techniques, and an improved understanding of expected outcomes. The objective of surgery for ROP-related detachments is to normalize the anatomy as much as possible in order to maximize visual potential. For macula-sparing (stage 4A) retinal detachments, the goal of surgical intervention is to achieve total retinal reattachment while preserving an undistorted posterior pole and a clear lens. Surgery for more advanced ROP detachments is performed to reattach as much of the retina as is possible with the functional goal of achieving ambulatory vision.

Anatomy of ROP-Related Retinal Detachments

Retinal detachments in ROP are generally preceded by fibrous proliferation and contraction of neovascularization along the ridge and into the overlying vitreous. The configuration of the ROP detachment depends on the vectors of vitreoretinal traction and their relationship to the ridge. Tractional forces can be oriented in the following ways:

1. Circumferential (Fig. 4.1a). Circumferential tractional vectors are intrinsic to the ridge itself, and cannot be removed surgically. Localized circumferential traction can result in a radial fold.
2. Ridge to lens (Fig. 4.1b). This antero-posterior vector extends between the midperipheral lens and the ridge

I. De la Huerta · A. Capone Jr (✉)
William Beaumont Hospital, Royal Oak, MI, USA
e-mail: acaponejr@arcpc.net

R. V. P. Chan (ed.), *Pediatric Retinal Diseases*, Retina Atlas, https://doi.org/10.1007/978-981-19-1364-8_4

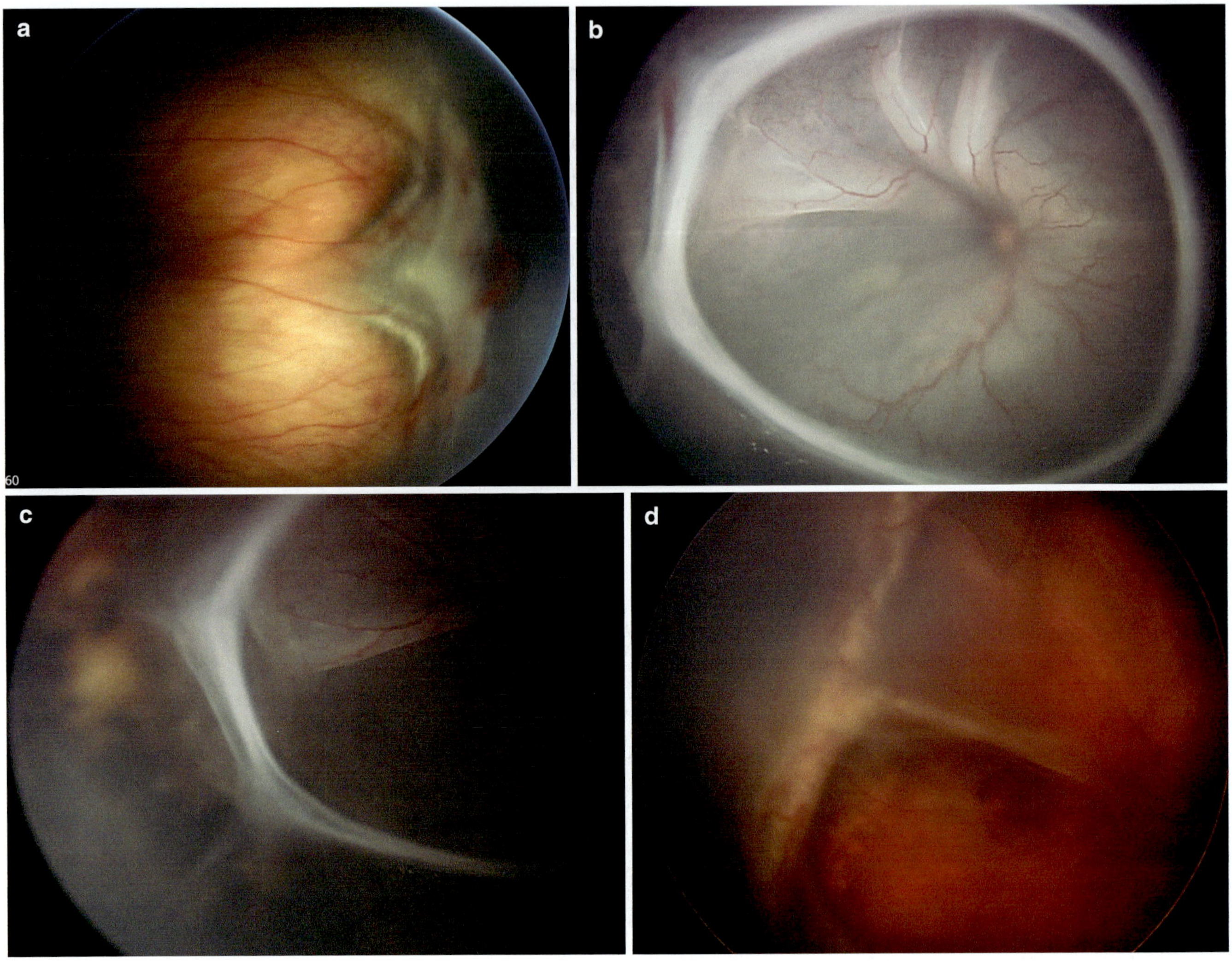

Fig. 4.1 (**a**) Circumferential contraction of proliferation intrinsic to the ridge results in a radial fold. (**b**) Tractional vectors extend anteriorly from the ridge toward the lens in an anteriorly open posteriorly open-funnel detachment. (**c**) Traction extends from the elevated ridge toward the retina just anterior to it. (**d**) A stalk-like band of proliferation exerts traction from the disc to the ridge

circumferentially in a purse-string pattern that draws the retina anteriorly and centrally.

3. Ridge to ciliary body. An organized vitreous sheet originating from the ridge extends anteriorly, pulling the ridge toward the ciliary processes.
4. Ridge to ridge. This tractional vector originates from the ridge and extends across to the contralateral ridge.
5. Ridge to peripheral retina (Fig. 4.1c).
6. Ridge to disc. Tractional vectors between the disc and the ridge can be of three types:
   (a) A stalk-like vitreous band that extends from the disc to the ridge, seen in eyes where the ridge is equatorial (Fig. 4.1d).
   (b) An epiretinal sheet tightly adherent to the retinal surface, that extends from the disc to the ridge where the ridge is posterior to the equator.
   (c) A transvitreal sheet extending from ridge to ridge and connected to the disc, typically seen in eyes where the ridge is anterior to the equator.

The overall configuration of an ROP-related retinal detachment is determined by the combination of the multiple tractional vectors present and by the location of the ridge or area of contracting neovascularization.

Surgical Goals

The goal of surgical intervention for ROP-related retinal detachments varies with the extent and severity of the detachment. The goals for macula-sparing retinal detachment (stage 4A ROP) are total retinal reattachment with an undis-

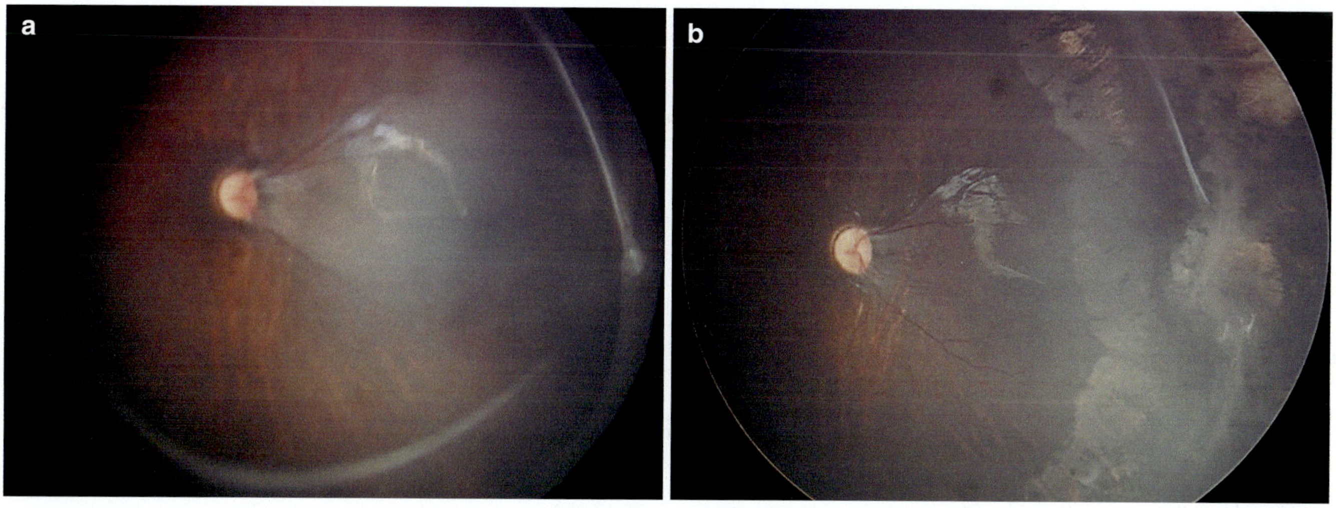

Fig. 4.2 (**a**) Stage 4B ROP-related tractional retinal detachment prior to surgery demonstrating subretinal fluid in the macula and temporal retina, with traction on the temporal ridge. (**b**) Resolved temporal stage 4B ROP-related tractional retinal detachment seen in Fig 4.3a following lens-sparing vitreous surgery

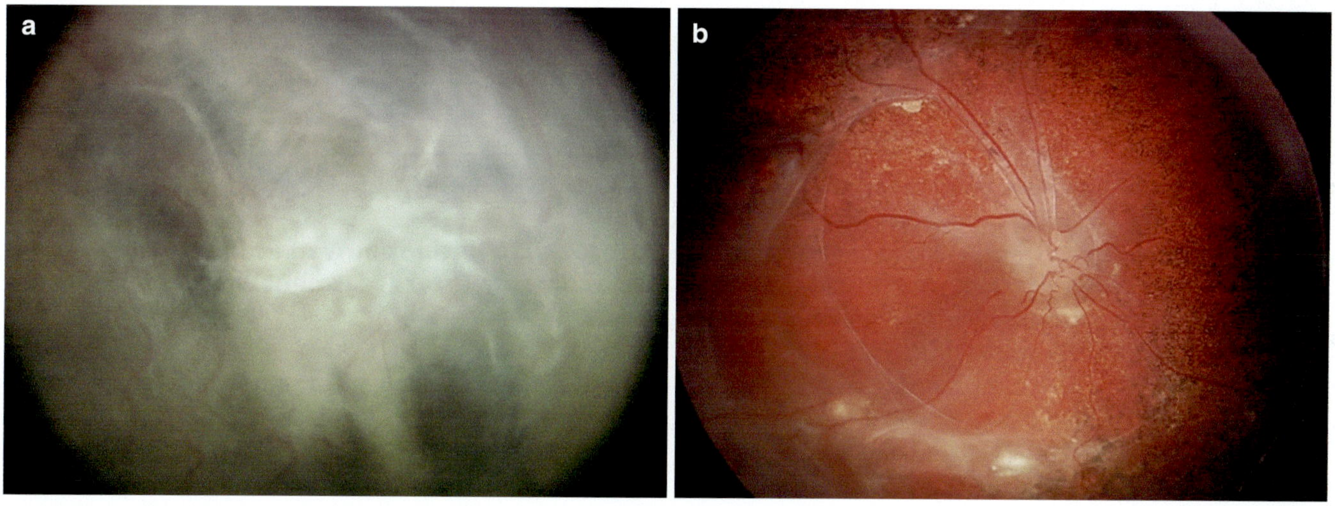

Fig. 4.3 (**a**) Stage 5 ROP-related tractional retinal detachment with retrolental fibroplasia prior to surgery. (**b**) Attached posterior retina in the eye seen in Fig. 4.4a following lensectomy and vitrectomy

torted posterior pole and lens preservation. In experienced centers, this outcome is achieved in over 80% of eyes with stage 4A ROP (Capone and Trese 2001; Hubbard III et al. 2004; Lakhanpal et al. 2005). Early functional outcomes appear encouraging as well, with two studies reporting average Snellen equivalent visual acuities (VA) of approximately 20/70 in patients tested with Teller acuity cards (average age 3–4 years) (Prenner et al. 2004; Lakhanpal et al. 2006).

The goal of surgery for macula-involving partial detachments (stage 4B ROP) is to minimize posterior pole distortion and prevent total retinal detachment (stage 5) (Fig. 4.2a, b). Vitrectomy directly addressing transvitreal traction can interrupt the progression to stage 5 ROP and may also improve macular dragging. Retinal attachment can be attained in a majority of cases and mean Snellen equivalent VA of 20/200 has been reported (Lakhanpal et al. 2006; El Rayes et al. 2008). The surgical goal for stage 5 ROP is to reattach as much of the retina as possible (Fig. 4.3a, b). The surgery involves addressing critical points of traction that can safely be removed without making a retinal break. A single iatrogenic break may lead to failure and subsequently to devastating proliferative vitreoretinopathy. Functionally, the goal of successful surgical therapy for stage 5 detachments is to preserve ambulatory vision.

Timing of Surgery

In general, earlier surgical intervention is preferred for ROP-related detachments as the prognosis for vision is best when the detachment is least extensive. Surgery for stage 4A ROP should be performed promptly to prevent macular detachment, particularly if the 4A detachment is located temporally. In eyes with stage 4 detachments and prior laser treatment, we recommend that surgery is typically done between 38 and 42 weeks postmenstrual age. Exceptions to this rule are stage 4 detachments in vascularly active eyes with marked plus disease that lack prior peripheral ablation. In such cases, there is a significant risk of uncontrollable bleeding during surgery, and it is better to treat the avascular peripheral retina first with laser. Eyes with stage 5 retinal detachments and significant vascular activity are similarly observed until 48–52 weeks postmenstrual age (Hartnett 2003).

Surgical Approach

Lens-Sparing Vitrectomy

Lens-sparing vitrectomy is the preferred approach for most stage 4 detachments and some open-funnel stage 5 detachments. This technique was initially reported for subtotal retinal detachments involving the macula, and has been associated with better postoperative VA compared to lensectomy with vitrectomy for stage 4b ROP (El Rayes et al. 2008). A two-port approach using infusing instruments such as an irrigating light pipe, pic, or spatula may be used. Alternatively an infusion can be placed through the pars plicata for a three-port approach. Vitrectomy is performed, addressing tractional vectors from the ridge to the lens, to the contralateral ridge, to the disc and to the peripheral retina. When this dissection is complete a fluid–air exchange is performed. The retina is not forced to reattach during the fluid–air exchange, as it will eventually reattach during the postoperative period if the vitreoretinal traction has been removed. The sclerotomies are closed. Subretinal fluid is gradually reabsorbed over weeks to months in the postoperative period.

Lensectomy and Vitrectomy

The presence of substantial retrolenticular fibrovascular proliferation in most stage 5 and some stage 4B-related retinal detachments typically requires combined lens removal and bimanual vitrectomy. The eye is entered at the limbus. Infusing instruments may be used in a two-port approach, or an infusion can be placed through the limbus inferiorly for a three-port approach. A partial iridectomy is typically performed to minimize reproliferation along the posterior iris and to improve visualization. Lensectomy is performed, followed by bimanual dissection to free the retina from traction as much as possible.

Some stage 5 eyes demonstrate shallowing of the anterior chamber with lens-cornea touch resulting in central corneal opacification. The surgical management of these cases requires a staged approach (Yonekawa et al. 2017a). The first stage procedure involves entering the eye at the nasal limbus with a butterfly needle that allows both infusion of fluid to maintain the anterior chamber and lysis of posterior synechiae. The vitreous cutter is then inserted through a temporal limbal incision into the crystalline lens, and lens material is aspirated to deepen the anterior chamber. Further synechiolysis and a partial iridectomy are then performed, followed by removal of the remaining lens material and capsule. After this first procedure, the cornea is allowed several weeks to clear sufficiently for the second stage: posterior segment surgery. The approach allows surgical intervention for stage 5 eyes with late presentation that are usually considered inoperable due to their corneal status.

Advanced Techniques

Approach to Retinopathy of Prematurity Detachments After Treatment with Anti-VEGF Agents

Two novel configurations of tractional retinal detachment following anti-VEGF therapy for ROP have recently been described (Yonekawa et al. 2017b). The prepapillary configuration is a posterior tractional detachment centered on the disc and caused by prepapillary hyaloidal contraction primarily in eyes where vascularization ended in posterior zone I at the time of anti-VEGF administration (Fig. 4.4). The circumferential configuration is a tight circular tractional detachment that may be caused by circumferential contraction of flat peripheral neovascularization (Fig. 4.5). In these cases, the surgical approach requires methodical delamination of the organized posterior hyaloid from the surface of the retina without creating iatrogenic breaks. Combining 23- or 25-gauge cannula-based instrumentation with introduction of a 27-gauge vitreous cutter to enter tighter planes may be useful in select cases (Yonekawa et al. 2016).

Enzymatic Vitreolysis

The stronger vitreoretinal adhesion in pediatric vitreoretinopathies such as ROP can lead to a more difficult vitreous

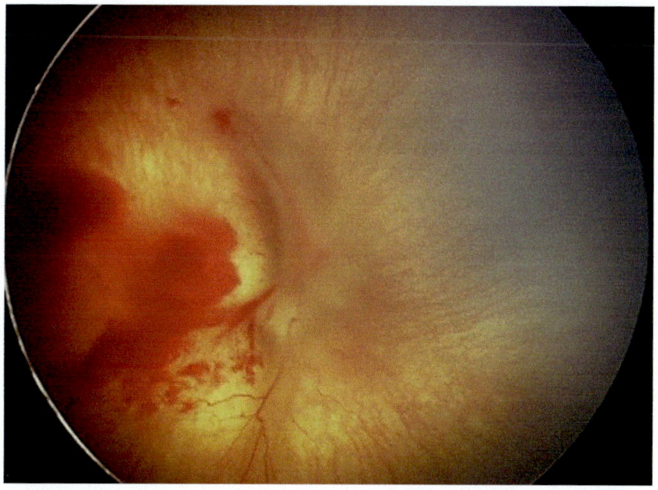

Fig. 4.4 Anti-VEGF-associated prepapillary tractional retinal detachment in ROP

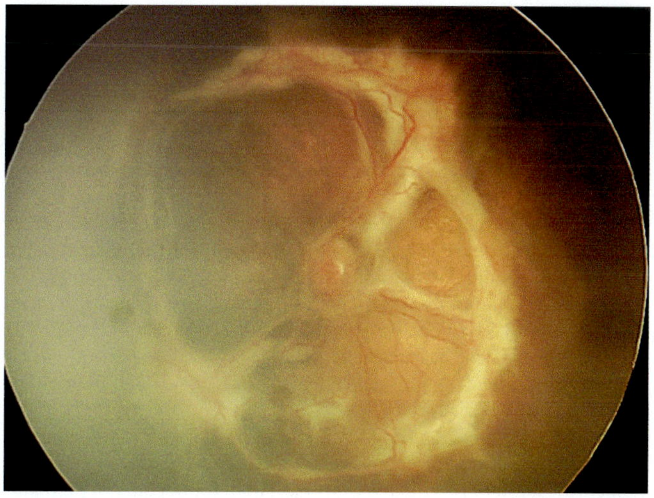

Fig. 4.5 Anti-VEGF-associated circumferential tractional retinal detachment in ROP

separation process during surgical vitrectomy. Although a Weiss ring may be apparent during attempted hyaloidal separation, the separation is likely to be lamellar, with residual vitreous left on the retinal surface. Retinal detachments in pediatric vitreoretinopathies often require adequate removal of layers of organized vitreous in order to achieve reattachment. Both autologous plasmin enzyme and ocriplasmin (Jetrea®; Thrombogenics, Leuven, Belgium) have been used as a pharmacologic vitreolysis agent to facilitate the induction of posterior vitreous detachment (PVD) during vitrectomy. Retrospective case series on the use of autologous plasmin lacked a control arm, but did demonstrate an acceptable safety profile, and autologous plasmin appeared to augment vitreous separation in ROP surgery (Wu et al. 2008; Wong and Capone 2013; Joshi et al. 2006). Ocriplasmin is a recombinant form of plasmin shown to be superior to placebo in resolving vitreomacular traction and in closing macular holes in adults (Stalmans et al. 2012). Ocriplasmin demonstrated no significant benefit compared to placebo in PVD induction during vitrectomy in a prospective randomized study of pediatric vitreoretinopathies, including ROP (Drenser et al. 2016). The small size of the study and the variety and complexity of the surgical cases limited the analysis. In general, the ability to dissociate the hyaloid from the retina with less mechanical force is advantageous. Additional studies focusing on specific retinal diseases and stages are needed to determine the role of these agents in vitrectomy surgery for ROP detachments.

Adult Retinopathy of Prematurity

Patients with regressed ROP continue to be at risk for vitreoretinal sequelae. The mechanism underlying late posterior segment disease is the persistence of abnormal vitreoretinal traction. Vitreous hemorrhage, retinal tears, and retinal detachments are some of the late sequelae of ROP in children and adults, prompting the need for lifelong monitoring (Kaiser et al. 2001; Spirn et al. 2006). Rhegmatogenous retinal detachments in adults with regressed ROP are challenging to repair due to atrophy of the peripheral retina and abnormalities of the vitreoretinal interface, especially over formerly avascular areas. Scleral buckling with additional support provided at the vitreous base, which is often posteriorly displaced, or a combination of vitrectomy with scleral buckling, may improve surgical success.

References

Banach MJ, Ferrone PJ, Trese MT. A comparison of dense versus less dense diode laser photocoagulation patterns for threshold retinopathy of prematurity. Ophthalmology. 2000;107:324–7.

Capone A, Trese MT. Lens-sparing vitreous surgery for tractional stage 4A retinopathy of prematurity retinal detachments. Ophthalmology. 2001;108:2068–70.

Cryotherapy for Retinopathy of Prematurity Cooperative Group. Multicenter trial of cryotherapy for retinopathy of prematurity. Preliminary results. Arch Ophthalmol. 1988;106:471–9.

Cryotherapy for Retinopathy of Prematurity Cooperative Group. The natural ocular outcome of premature birth and retinopathy. Status at 1 year. Arch Ophthalmol. 1994;112:903–12.

Drenser KA, Trese MT, Capone A. Aggressive posterior retinopathy of prematurity. Retina. 2010;30:S37–40.

Drenser K, Girach A, Capone A. A randomized, placebo-controlled study of intravitreal ocriplasmin in pediatric patients scheduled for vitrectomy. Retina. 2016;36:565–75.

Early Treatment for Retinopathy of Prematurity Cooperative Group. Revised indications for the treatment of retinopathy of prematurity: results of the early treatment for retinopathy of prematurity randomized trial. Arch Ophthalmol. 2003;121:1684–94.

El Rayes EN, Vinekar A, Capone A Jr. Three-year anatomic and visual outcomes after vitrectomy for stage 4B retinopathy of prematurity. Retina. 2008;28:568–72.

Funk M, Kriechbaum K, Prager F, et al. Intraocular concentrations of growth factors and cytokines in retinal vein occlusion and the effect of therapy with bevacizumab. Invest Ophthalmol Vis Sci. 2009;50:1025–32.

Good WV, Early Treatment for Retinopathy of Prematurity Cooperative Group. Final results of the early treatment for retinopathy of prematurity randomized trial. Trans Am Ophthalmol Soc. 2004;102:233–48.

Gunn DJ, Cartwright DW, Cole GA. Prevalence and outcomes of laser treatment of aggressive posterior retinopathy of prematurity. Clin Exp Ophthalmol. 2014;42:459–65.

Hartnett ME. Features associated with surgical outcome in patients with stages 4 and 5 retinopathy of prematurity. Retina. 2003;23:322–9.

Hubbard GB III, Cherwick DH, Burian G. Lens-sparing vitrectomy for stage 4 retinopathy of prematurity. Ophthalmology. 2004;111(12):2274–7.

Joshi MM, Ciaccia S, Trese MT, Capone A. Posterior hyaloid contracture in pediatric vitreoretinopathies. Retina. 2006;26:S38–41.

Kaiser RS, Trese MT, Williams GA, et al. Adult retinopathy of prematurity. Outcomes of rhegmatogenous and retinal tears. Ophthalmology. 2001;108:1647–53.

Lakhanpal RR, Sun RL, Albini TA, et al. Anatomic success rate after 3-port lens-sparing vitrectomy in stage 4A or 4B retinopathy of prematurity. Ophthalmology. 2005;112:1569–73.

Lakhanpal RR, Sun RL, Albini TA, et al. Visual outcomes after 3-port lens-sparing vitrectomy in stage 4 retinopathy of prematurity. Arch Ophthalmol. 2006;124:675–9.

Prenner JL, Capone A Jr, Trese MT. Visual outcomes after lens-sparing vitrectomy for stage 4A retinopathy of prematurity. Ophthalmology. 2004;111(12):2271–3.

Rezai KA, Eliott D, Ferrone PJ, Kim RW. Near confluent laser photocoagulation for the treatment of threshold retinopathy of prematurity. Arch Ophthalmol. 2005;123:621–6.

Sato T, Kusaka S, Shimojo H, Fujikado T. Simultaneous analyses of vitreous levels of 27 cytokines in eyes with retinopathy of prematurity. Ophthalmology. 2009;116:2165–9.

Snyder LL, Garcia-Gonzalez JM, Shapiro MJ, Blair MP. Very late reactivation of retinopathy of prematurity after monotherapy with intravitreal bevacizumab. Ophthalmic Surg Lasers Imaging Retina. 2016;47:280–3.

Spirn MJ, Lynn MJ, Hubbard GB 3rd. Vitreous hemorrhage in children. Ophthalmology. 2006;113:848–52.

Stalmans P, Benz MS, Gandorfer A, et al. Enzymatic vitreolysis with ocriplasmin for vitreomacular traction and macular holes: MIVI-TRUST study group. N Engl J Med. 2012;16:606–15.

Wong SC, Capone A. Microplasmin (ocriplasmin) in pediatric vitreoretinal surgery: update and review. Retina. 2013;33:339–48.

Wu WC, Drenser KA, Lai M, Capone A, Trese MT. Plasmin enzyme-assisted vitrectomy for primary and reoperated eyes with stage 5 retinopathy of prematurity. Retina. 2008;28:S75–80.

Yonekawa Y, Thanos A, Abbey AM, et al. Hybrid 25- and 27-gauge vitrectomy for complex vitreoretinal surgery. Ophthalmic Surg Lasers Imaging Retina. 2016;47:352–5.

Yonekawa Y, Thomas BJ, Thanos A, et al. The cutting edge of retinopathy of prematurity care: expanding the boundaries of diagnosis and treatment. Retina. 2017a; [Epub ahead of print].

Yonekawa Y, Wu WC, Nitulescu CE, et al. Progressive retinal detachment in infants with retinopathy of prematurity treated with intravitreal bevacizumab or ranibizumab. Retina 2017b; [Epub ahead of print].

5 Atypical Retinopathy of Prematurity

Tapas Ranjan Padhi and Subhadra Jalali

ROP in Big Babies

ROP is described as a disease exclusively seen in premature born babies, especially those with low birth weight. The National ROP screening guidelines regarding Gestational age (GA) and Birth weight (BW) are variable across countries. However, most criteria also include babies "beyond the criteria" such as "babies where Pediatrician has concerns," "sickness criteria," or "stormy neonatal course." This invariably brings in late pre-terms and sometimes term babies and heavier babies with higher birth weight. The ROP characteristics of few such babies have been reported and are collectively termed here as "ROP in Big babies."

ROP in Near Term and Big Babies Is Rarely Reported

A Series of four babies (Fig. 5.1a–d) with GA 36–39 weeks and, Birth weight 2.4–3.0 kg. were reported (Padhi et al. 2015). ROP Screening was done due to multiple systemic problems during neonatal period. Fundus evaluation showed Zone III disease in three babies and Early stage of APROP in Zone II in one baby.

In the study on universal newborn screening (Goyal et al. 2018) using wide field digital images, additional term babies with ROP-like lesions were seen (Fig. 5.2). Two babies showed retinal ridge akin to ROP despite being term with birth weight >2.5 kg. The ridge regressed in one, and the other child was lost to follow up. We were careful and cross-checked GA and BW from multiple sources and ruled out ROP mimickers like Familial exudative Vitreoretinopathy (FEVR), incontinentia pigmenti and primary bone marrow failure disorders.

Aggressive Posterior ROP in Bigger Babies

This is extremely rare, but big babies can also present with atypical aggressive posterior ROP (APROP) (Fig. 5.3). This baby had GA 35 weeks and BW 3600 g with the non-diabetic mother affected by Pregnancy-induced hypertension. Baby presented at a post-menstrual age (PMA) of 39 weeks and weighed 4200 g at examination. Marked dilatation and tortuosity of the retinal vessels with shunting at multiple levels with flat new vessels within vascularized retina were noted. There was a good response to prompt confluent laser (Fig. 5.4).

Zone Half-APROP (APROP with Vascularization Not Even Reached Near Fovea) and Posterior Zone 1 ROP Variant

Numerous clinicians, especially from India, have reported severe posterior disease where the vascular growth from the disc consists of only sparse vessels and the posterior pole vessels have not even reached the foveal area. Results of laser alone are not encouraging (Katoch et al. 2019). Often though not always they develop APROP configuration. The baby here had GA 25 weeks, BW 650 g and was born with assisted fertilization. Neonatal period was significant for respiratory distress, anemia, apnea, and multiple blood transfusions. At first screening at 28 weeks PMA, baby had Zone I very immature retina, only four tiny vessels were seen close

T. R. Padhi
Anant Bajaj Retina Institute, Pediatric Retina Services, Dalmia Newborn Eye Health Alliance (NEHA) and Miriam Hyman Children Eye Care Center (MHCECC), L V Prasad Eye Institute, Bhubaneswar, Odisha, India
e-mail: tapas@lvpei.org

S. Jalali (✉)
Anant Bajaj Retina Institute, Srimati Kanuri Santhamma Centre for Vitreoretinal Diseases, L V Prasad Eye Institute, Hyderabad, Telangana, India

Jasti V ramanamma Childrens' Eye Care Centre, L V Prasad Eye Institute, Hyderabad, Telangana, India
e-mail: Subhadra@lvpei.org

R. V. P. Chan (ed.), *Pediatric Retinal Diseases*, Retina Atlas, https://doi.org/10.1007/978-981-19-1364-8_5

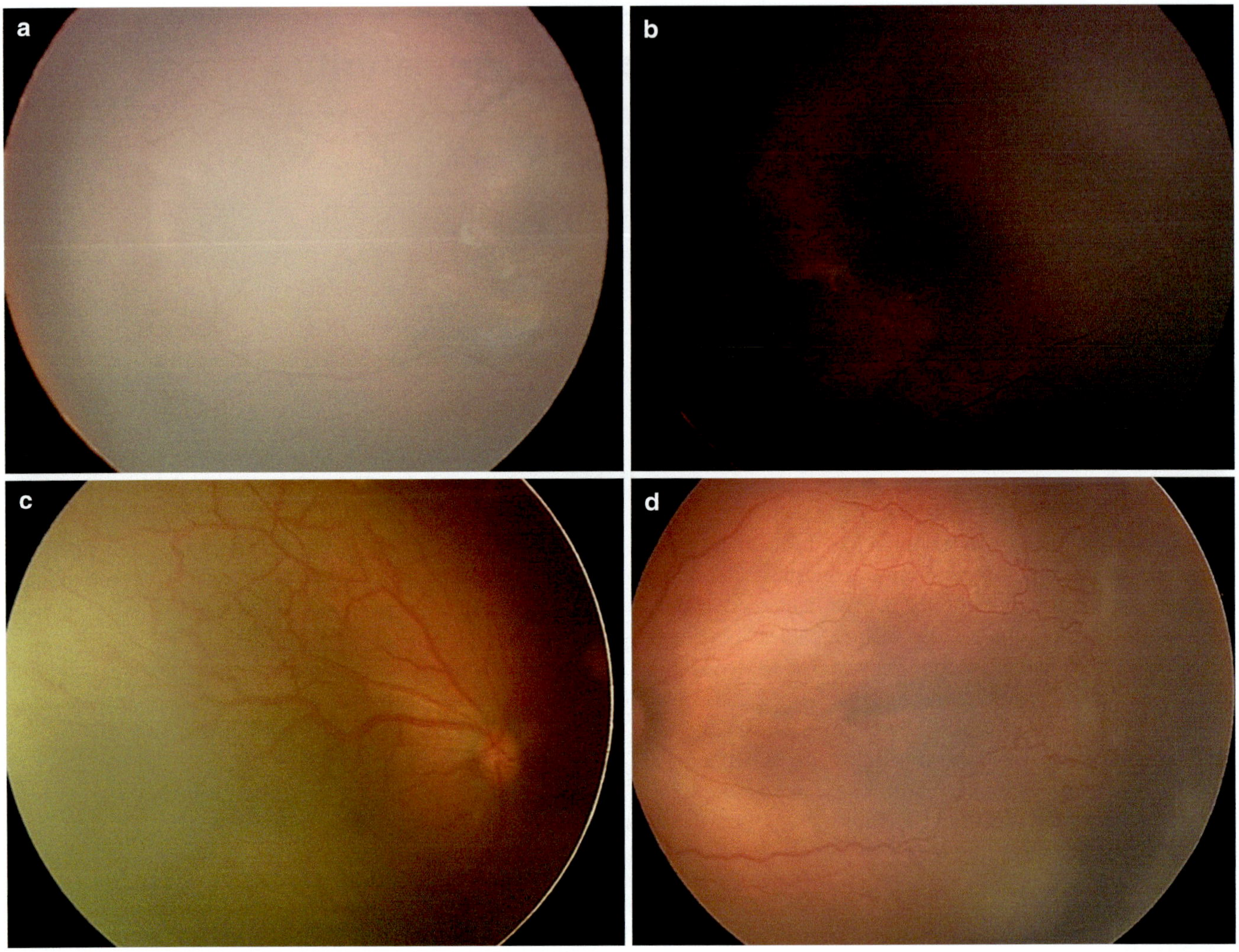

Fig. 5.1 (**a**–**d**) Composite fundus images of a series of a series of three babies (**a**–**d**) with GA 36–39 weeks and birth weight 2.4–3.0 kg (**a** and **b**). Fundus picture of right and left eyes of case 1 showing a ridge in zone III. (**c**) Right eye of case 2 with marked dilatation and tortuosity of retinal vessels in all quadrant involving posterior pole with shunting at multiple levels suggestive of aggressive posterior ROP in Zone I. (**d**) Fundus picture of the left eye (case 3) showing a ridge in zone III [Image taken with permission from the article published by the authors in 'Eye' (Padhi et al. 2015)]

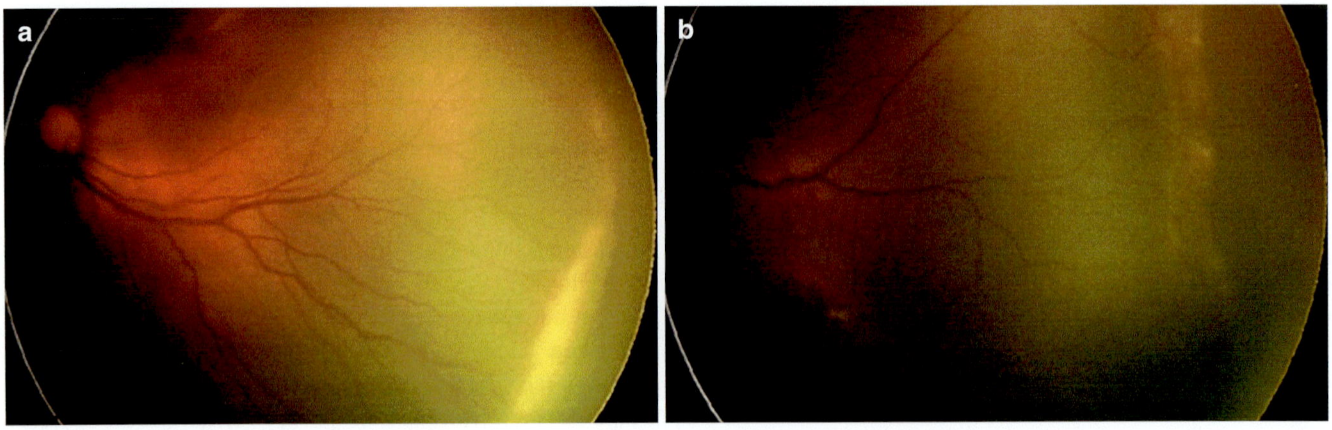

Fig. 5.2 (**a**, **b**) Fundus picture of left eyes of two full-term babies with birth weight more than 2.5 kg were found to have a ridge in zone II during a routine newborn eye screening within 1 week of birth. The fundus examination of the parents and siblings was unremarkable. The ridge regressed spontaneously with time and fundus picture of the parents and siblings were unremarkable

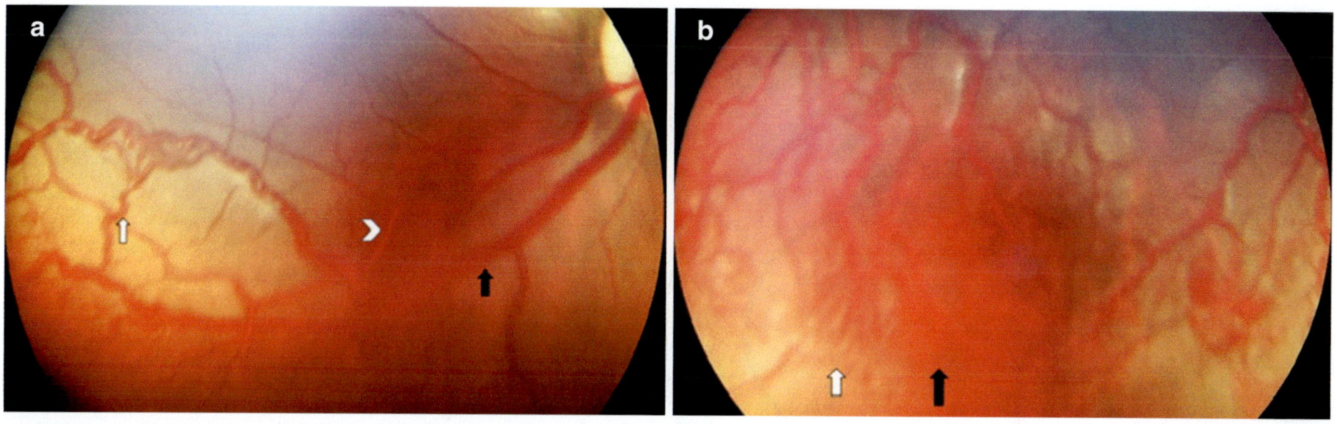

Fig. 5.3 (**a**, **b**) Fundus picture of a baby with Gestational age 35 week and birth weight 3600 g showing marked dilatation (black arrow) and tortuosity of retinal vessels with shunting (white arrow head) at multiple levels and flat new vessels suggestive of aggressive retinopathy of prematurity

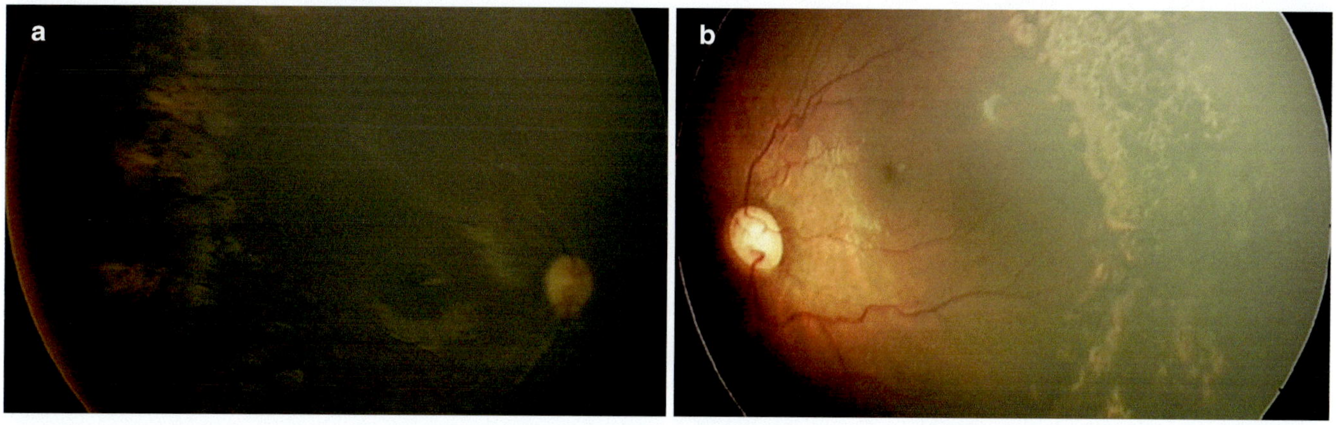

Fig. 5.4 (**a**, **b**) Fundus pictures of the right and left eyes of the same baby as in Fig. 5.3, 1 month post laser showing complete regression

to the disc (picture not available, retinal drawing shown Fig. 5.5).

At PMA 31 weeks, severe APROP and underdeveloped foveal architecture was noted (Fig. 5.6). The baby was treated with off-label IVB (Intravitreal Bevacizumab) in both eyes. Figures 5.7, 5.8 and 5.9 show the serial fundus changes on close follow-up.

Hybrid ROP

APROP and staged ROP have very distinct vascular patterns and clinical courses (Agarwal and Jalali 2018). The Hybrid ROP has mixed vascular pattern (Fig. 5.10). It is characterized by vascular pattern that has both APROP features (posterior location and abnormal pattern of looped vessels having variable-sized pockets or islands of avascular retina with no definitive ridge) and staged ROP features (normal vascular pattern of dichotomously branching vascular growth at the end of which the vessels proliferate but do not move forwards giving classical stages 1–3 at well-defined junction of vascular and avascular retina).It is seen in bigger babies, often administered subnormal neonatal and perinatal care. The four-lobed topography may be absent, severe disease is quite often present nasally also, and the posterior retinal vascularization is better grown than in APROP. Ridge tissue is variable (Sanghi et al. 2012). Depending on extent and time point when baby is first seen, these eyes could respond to laser alone or a combination of laser and Intravitreal Anti-VEGF injection.

Bleb-Like Posterior Combined Tractional and Exudative Retinal Detachment in ROP

This variant is characterized by combined tractional and exudative retinal detachment confined to posterior pole area, obscuring the disc and macula (Patel et al. 2020). There is attached completely avascular peripheral retina. The detached retina has scanty retinal vessels and larger proportion of fibrous component. The elevated area is four lobed, with kidney-shaped bleb-like configuration (Fig. 5.11). This

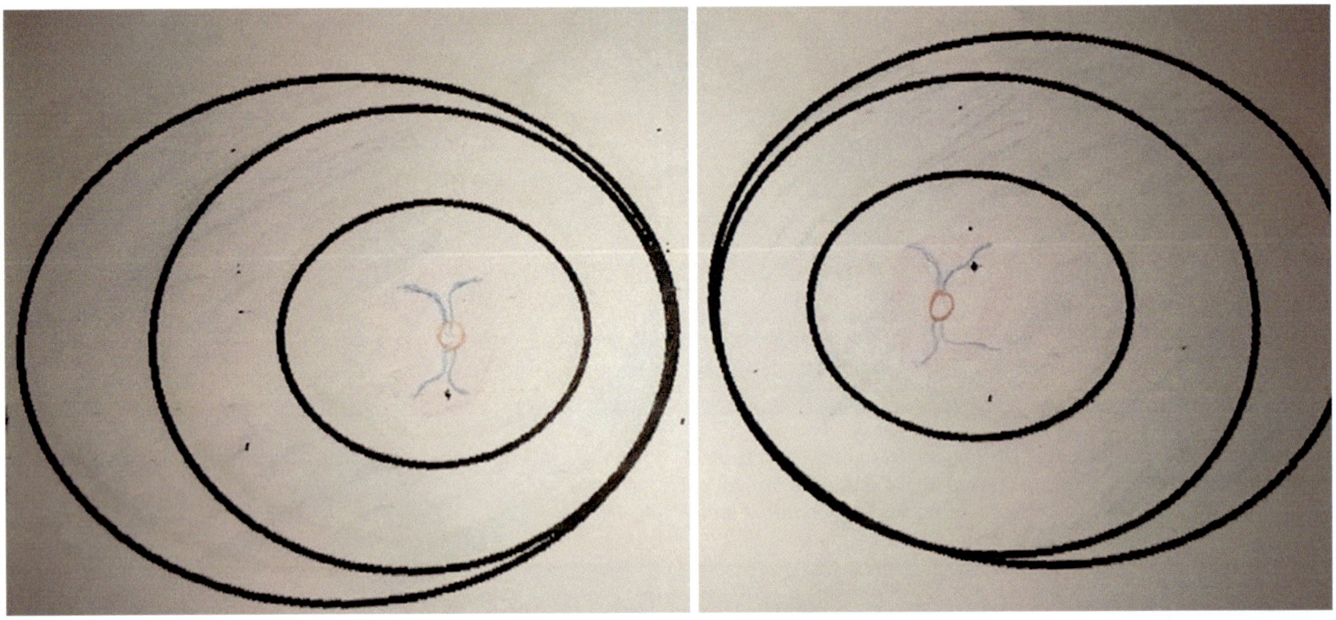

Fig. 5.5 Freehand drawing showing immature retina in zone I posterior. The blood vessels were very thin and hardly extended beyond posterior zone I

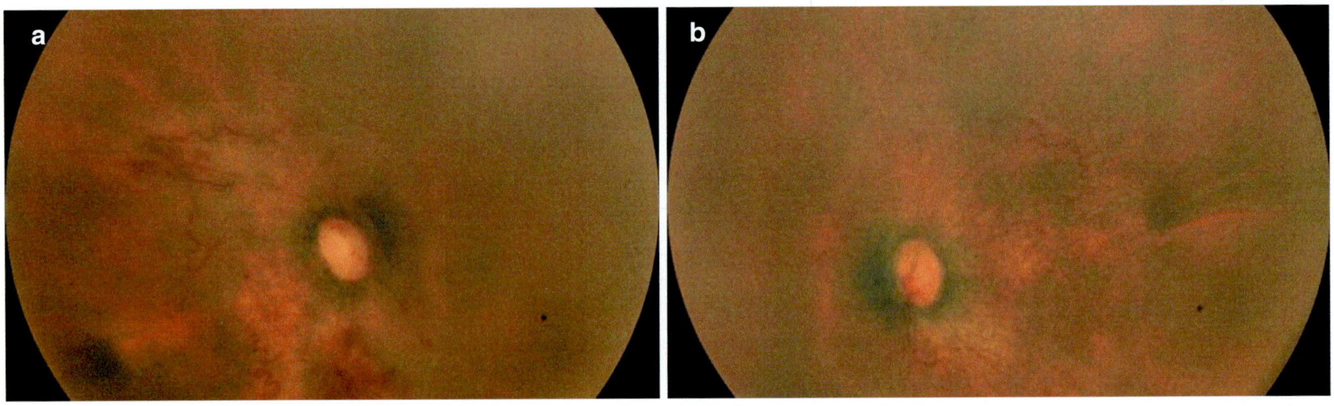

Fig. 5.6 (**a**, **b**) Fundus images of both eyes of the same baby at 31 weeks of post-menstrual age showing few loops of dilated and tortuous blood vessels around optic disc with foveal immaturity. The blood vessels were hardly extending beyond one disc diameter from the disc nasally

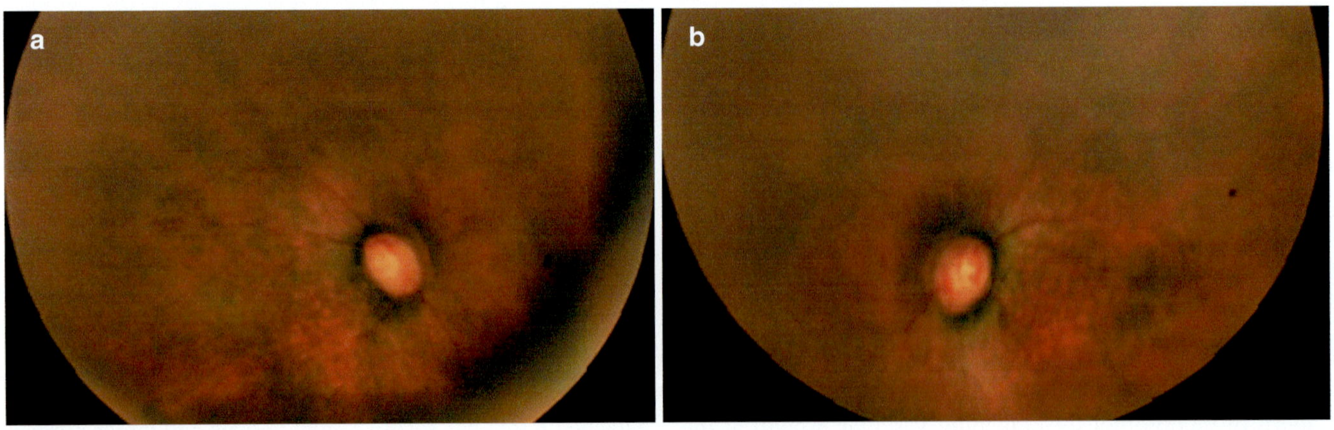

Fig. 5.7 (**a**, **b**) Fundus picture of both eyes of the same baby at 32 weeks of post-menstrual age (1 week post intravitreal bevacizumab) showing marked reduction in the dilatation and tortuosity with very slow vascular growth

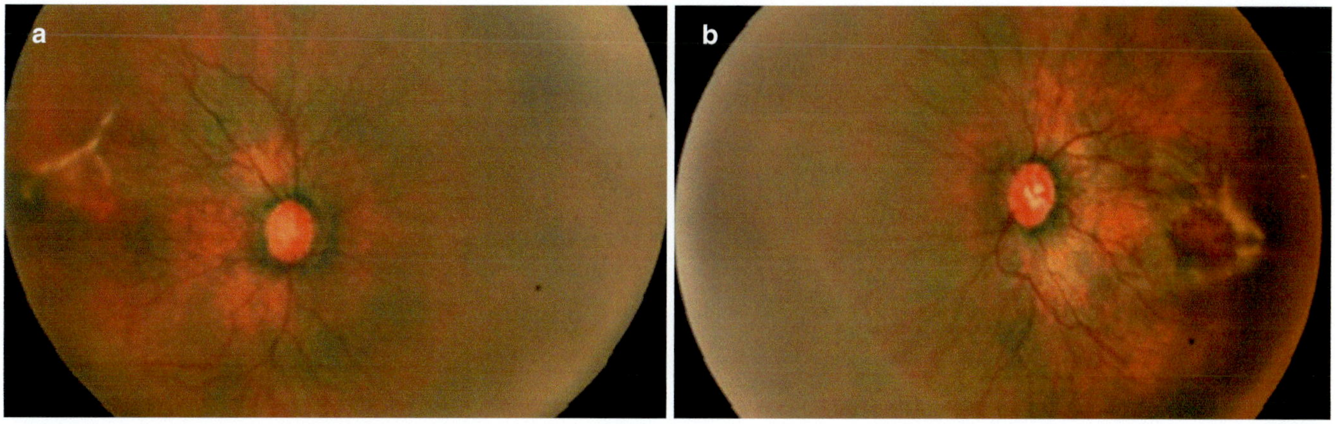

Fig. 5.8 (**a**, **b**) Fundus picture of both eyes of the same baby at post-menstrual age of 36 weeks, showing some growth of vasculature and absent ridge tissue

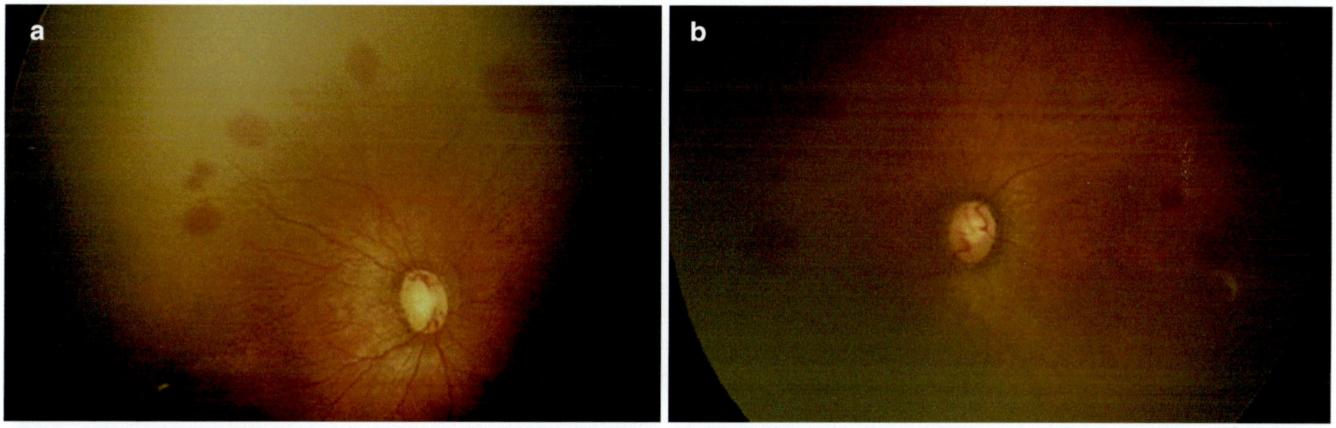

Fig. 5.9 (**a**, **b**) Fundus picture of both eyes of the same baby at a post-menstrual age of 37 weeks, recurrence of disease manifested by wreath of deep retinal hemorrhages at the leading edge of vascularised retina. A second dose of intravitreal bevacizumab was given. Note foveal architecture started to develop. These eyes usually need additional laser for repeated recurrences

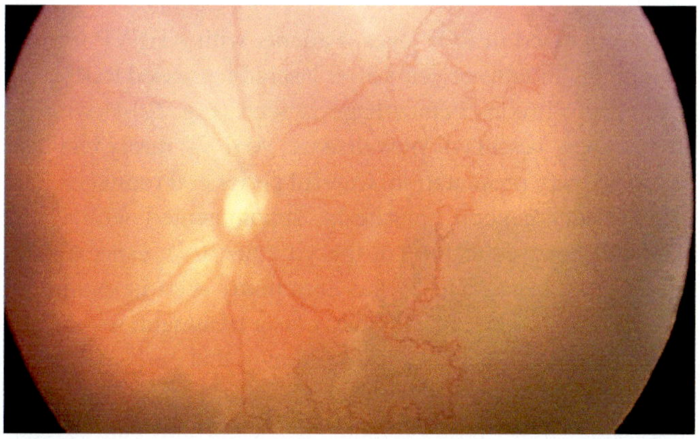

Fig. 5.10 Fundus picture of the right eye showing dilatation and tortuosity along with arteriovenous shunting within zone I at multiple levels suggestive of hybrid ROP. There are pockets of avascular retina within the vascular loops

responds only in some eyes to combined therapy of laser, IVB and Vitrectomy carried out in very quick succession, often within 2–4 days (Fig. 5.12).

Exudative Retinal Detachment as an Initial Presentation in ROP

Retinal detachment in ROP is predominantly tractional in nature. Rarely severe ROP can be associated with some peripheral exudation or exudative retinal detachment in periphery can develop after the use of excessive strong laser burns. Primary exudative retinal detachment especially involving large parts of retina at the initial presentation itself is quite atypical (Jayanna et al. 2020).

Case: GA 30 weeks, birth weight 1500 g seen at 34 weeks PMA. Baby had been treated for necrotizing enterocolitis

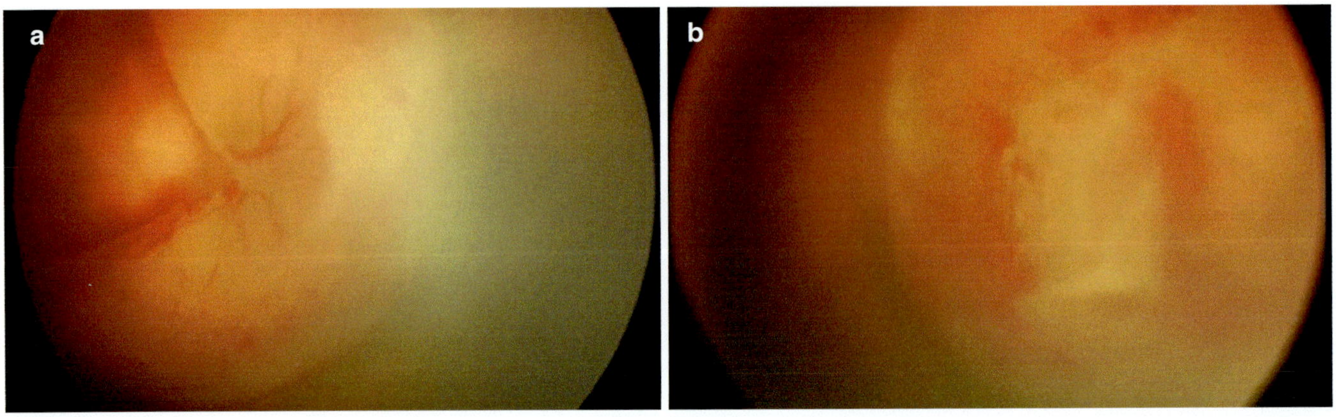

Fig. 5.11 (**a**, **b**) RetCam fundus images of the right (**a**) and left eyes (**b**) of a baby at 35 weeks of post-menstrual age. He had a gestational age of 28 weeks, birth weight 1135 g and was on oxygen supplementation for 30 days. Both eyes showed fibrovascular proliferation and an indistinct retinal vasculature sitting on the top of a bleb-shaped retinal detachment in either eye. The eyes were treated with intravitreal bevacizumab (day 1), laser (day 4) and vitrectomy (day 9)

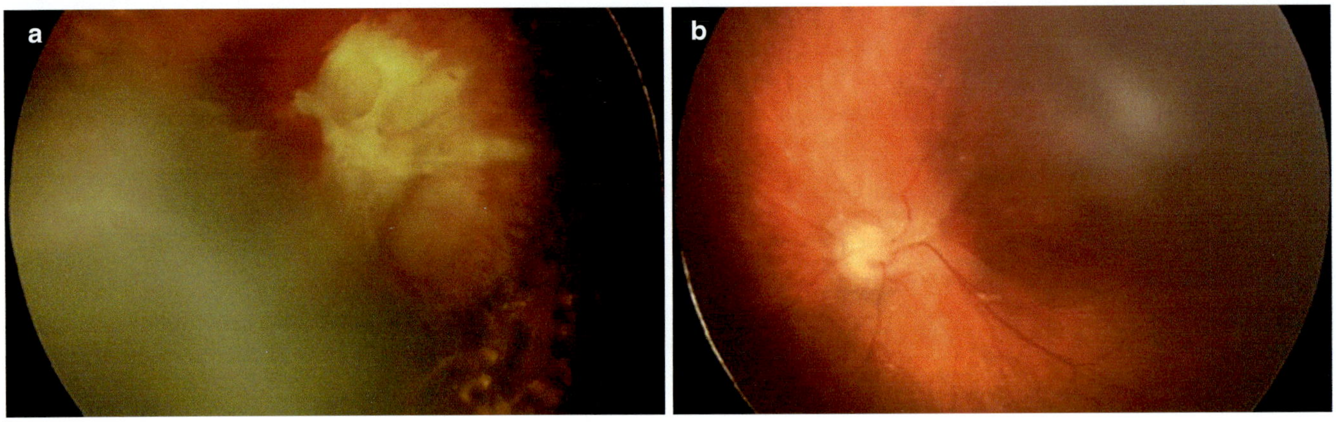

Fig. 5.12 (**a**, **b**) Final outcome of the eyes of the same baby shown in Fig. 5.11. While the left eye did well after single surgery (**b**), right eye required re-surgery twice once for persistent postoperative bleeding over the entire detached retina and later for progressive anteroposterior traction along anterior hyaloid (**a**)

and anemia. At presentation there was bilateral posterior exudative retinal detachment causing a macular fold, with APROP changes in posterior zone II (Fig. 5.13a). Right eye was treated with intravitreal bevacizumab (Fig. 5.13a) followed by laser. Post resolution, macular RPE changes were visible at the site of past exudation (Fig. 5.13b).

Anterior Hyaloidal Fibrovascular Proliferation in ROP

Anterior hyaloidal fibrovascular proliferation (AHFVP) characterized by new vessels and fibrous tissue proliferation at the vitreous base causing recurrent vitreous hemorrhage is not uncommon in vascular retinopathies like Diabetic retinopathy, Retinal vein occlusions and retinal vasculitis. It is not well recognized in ROP eyes. Patients with AHFVP usually present few months or years after lasered regressed ROP eyes. Late-onset vitreous hemorrhage is seen (Fig. 5.14) with no obvious new vessels or plus disease. AHFVP rarely can also be the primary presentation. Careful peripheral retinal examination under general anesthesia, supplemented with UBM reveals fibrovascular tufts at the vitreous base, especially in inferior half of the eye. It was commonly seen in extremely preterm babies who had very early laser treatment, within 2–3 weeks of birth. It is hypothesized that at that early PMA, the anterior retina grows after the initial laser had regressed the ROP. This "new" retina remains avascular and can develop ROP silently in the anterior most retina, without changes near the posterior pole. The condition responded very well to vitreous base transscleral cryotherapy with or without adjunct anti-VEGF injection or laser (Dave et al. 2004).

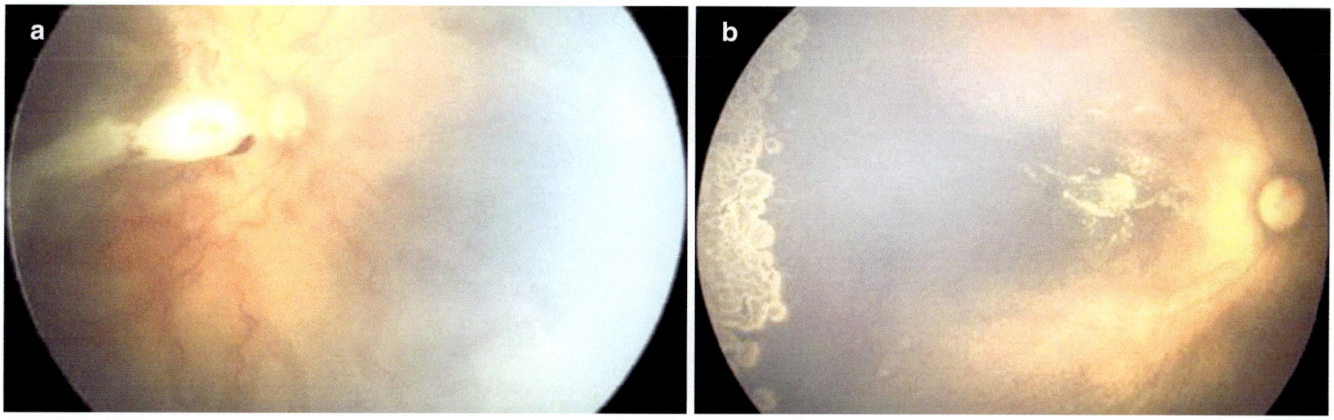

Fig. 5.13 (**a**, **b**) RetCam fundus images of the right eye (**a**) at presentation showing features of APROP and an exudative detachment causing a retinal fold at macula. The detachment and the retinopathy regressed well after a single intravitreal injection and laser photocoagulation (**b**)

Fig. 5.14 Fundus picture of a case of lasered and regressed ROP that presented with vitreous hemorrhages years after regression. There were no plus components or clinically obvious new vessels in the retina to count for vitreous hemorrhage

Summary Atypical presentations in ROP range from mild disease that regresses spontaneously to severe disease not responding to conventional laser therapy. The atypical patterns are seen both during the acute phase of the disease and also months or days after treatment. They could be unilateral, though commonly bilateral. A combination of various treatment modalities that are dictated by the clinical picture and extrapolating from typical ROP or other vascular retinopathies can give a direction to treatment modality.

Note This chapter describes the off-label use of intravitreal Bevacizumab.

Financial Disclosures Both the authors do not have any financial disclosures. The L V Prasad Eye Institute receives funding by Government and Non-Government agencies for expansion of various ROP programs. None of these are involved in current work.

References

Agarwal K, Jalali S. Classification of Retinopathy of prematurity: from then till now. Community Eye Health (South Asia ed). 2018;31(101):S4–7.

Dave VP, Jalali S, Rani PK, Padhi TR. Characteristics and outcomes of anterior hyaloidal fibrovascular proliferation in lasered Retinopathy of Prematurity. The Indian Twin cities retinopathy of prematurity study report number 4. Int Ophthalmol. 2004;34:511–7. https://doi.org/10.1007/s10792-013-9843-2.

Goyal P, Padhi TR, Das T, Pradhan L, Sutar S, Butola S, et al. Outcome of universal newborn eye screening with wide-field digital retinal image acquisition system: a pilot study. Eye. 2018;32:67–73. https://doi.org/10.1038/eye.2017.129.

Jayanna S, Agarwal K, Padhi TR, Jalali S. Exudative retinal detachment as an initial presentation in retinopathy of prematurity. JAAPOS. 2020;S1091-8531(20):30205–6. https://doi.org/10.1016/j.jaapos.2020.07.006.

Katoch D, Dogra MR, Agarwal K, Sanghi G, Samantha R, Handa S, et al. Posterior Zone 1 Retinopathy of prematurity; Spectrum of disease and outcome after laser treatment. Can J Ophthalmol. 2019;54:87–93. https://doi.org/10.1016/j.jcjo.2018.03.005.

Padhi TR, Rath S, Jalali S, Pradhan L, Kesarwani S, Nayak M, et al. Larger and near-term baby retinopathy: a rare case series. Eye (Lond). 2015;29(2):286–9. https://doi.org/10.1038/eye.2014.253.

Patel A, Padhy SK, Saoji K, Saldna M, Multani PK, Khals A, et al. Bleb-like posterior combined retinal detachment in severe Retinopathy of Prematurity: clinical characteristics, management challenges, and outcome. Eye. (2020). https://doi.org/10.1038/s41433-020-01223-0. Epub ahead of print.

Sanghi G, Dogra M, Katoch D, Guota A. A hybrid form of retinopathy of prematurity. Br J Ophthalmol. 2012;96:519–22. https://doi.org/10.1136/bjophthalmol-2011-300321.

Persistent Fetal Vasculature

6

Parag K. Shah, S. Prema, Parth Patil, and V. Narendran

Introduction

Persistent fetal vasculature (PFV) is an ocular disorder in which the fetal vasculature does not regress (Goldberg 1997) and is unilateral in about 90% of cases. PFV was first described by Reese (1955) when it was termed as persistent hyperplastic primary vitreous (PHPV). PFV has now been adopted as this addresses the fact that the persistent hyaloid vessels and tunica vascular lentis can persist and lead to a spectrum of structural changes within the eye (Goldberg 1997). The disease may manifest with having subtle changes with no visual disturbance to more severe forms of the condition developing phthisis bulbi or secondary glaucoma. In less severe forms of PFV, prompt diagnosis and early intervention with appropriate amblyopic therapy may result in good visual outcome.

Etiopathogenesis

Embryonic Development

The vitreous has three components: the primary, secondary, and tertiary vitreous.

The primary vitreous forms during the first month of fetal life in the space between the lens and the retina. It consists of mesodermally derived tissue, including the hyaloid vessels and its branches and a fibrillar meshwork. Remnants of the primitive hyaloid system often persist in small infants. Anteriorly (Mittendorf's dot behind the lens posterior pole), posteriorly (Bergmeister's papilla at the optic disc), or more extensively (hyaloid vessels).

The secondary vitreous or definitive adult vitreous forms during the second month of embryonic development and is composed of 99% of water bound with collagen and hyaluronic acid.

The tertiary vitreous develops during the fourth month of gestation and forms the zonules of Zinn which suspends the lens (Sebag 2000).

The fetal vasculature (primitive hyaloid system) is composed of two parts:

1. Anterior tunica vasculosa lentis. It is situated anteriorly encircling the lens. It has anterior and posterior divisions. The anterior division has additional attachments to the pupillary frill of the iris. The posterior division has additional attachments to the ciliary process and continues with the hyaloid artery posteriorly.
2. Posterior hyaloid artery. It is situated posteriorly behind the lens. The hyaloid vessel extends from the posterior surface of lens to the disc. The vasculature fills the vitreous cavity and has many attachments to the retinal surface.

This term PFV emphasizes the importance of both the anterior tunica vasculosa lentis and the persistent posterior hyaloid system and also represents the spectrum of structural changes which can present within the eye.

Normal Regression of Embryonic Vascular System (Sebag and Nguyen 2005)

During development, blood flow to the eye is through the hyaloid artery. At the 240-mm stage (seventh month) in the human, blood flow in the hyaloid artery ceases. Hyaloid vascular regression occurs in following manner:

The developing lens separates the fetal vasculature from vascular endothelial growth factor (VEGF) producing cells,

Supplementary Information The online version contains supplementary material available at [https://doi.org/10.1007/978-981-19-1364-8_6].

P. K. Shah (✉) · S. Prema · P. Patil · V. Narendran
Department of Pediatric Retina, Aravind Eye Hospital & Postgraduate Institute of Ophthalmology, Coimbatore, Tamil Nadu, India

R. V. P. Chan (ed.), *Pediatric Retinal Diseases*, Retina Atlas, https://doi.org/10.1007/978-981-19-1364-8_6

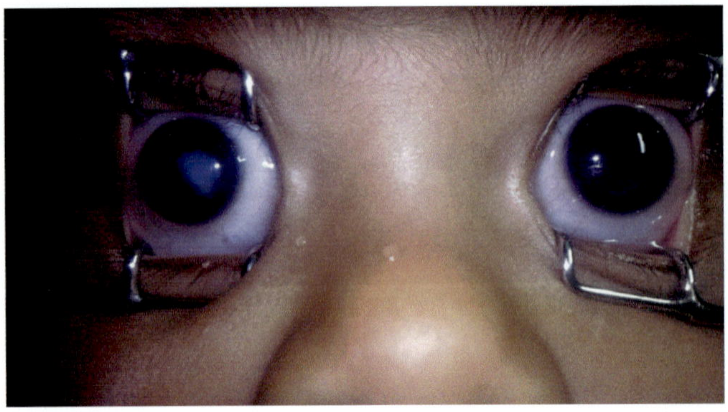

Fig. 6.1 Anterior PFV showing retrolental fibrovascular membrane in the right eye. The left eye is normal

inducing apoptosis. Meeson et al. (1996) proposed that there are actually two forms of apoptosis.

↓

The first form called initiating apoptosis results from macrophage induction of apoptosis in a single endothelial cell.

↓

The isolated dying endothelial cell projects into the capillary lumen and interferes with blood flow.

↓

This stimulates synchronous apoptosis of downstream endothelial cells called secondary apoptosis and ultimately causes obliteration of the vasculature.

No single gene is isolated with PFV. Association with pax6 gene is recently documented in optic nerve head anomalies which include PFV (Azuma et al. 2003). Linkage to 10q11-q21 has also been reported (Khaliq et al. 2001).

Clinical Features and Classification

There are three types of PFV:

1. *Anterior PFV:* It has predominant features of persistent anterior tunica vasculosa lentis without much or any posterior hyaloid component.
   (a) Presentation age 1–2 weeks with leukocoria. Leukocoria is the most common presentation of the disease. PFV is the second most common cause of leukocoria.
   (b) Microphthalmos.
   (c) Posterior lens opacity → cataract.
   (d) Retrolental fibrovascular membrane (varies in size from a small plaque to complete covering of posterior capsule of the lens (Fig. 6.1)). The tissue is thickest near the centre with associated vessels having radial pattern termed brittle star sign by Goldberg (1997)
   (e) Shallow anterior chamber → glaucoma.
   (f) Elongated ciliary process → hypotony.
   (g) Stalk extending from the posterior part of lens to the optic disc may not be present.

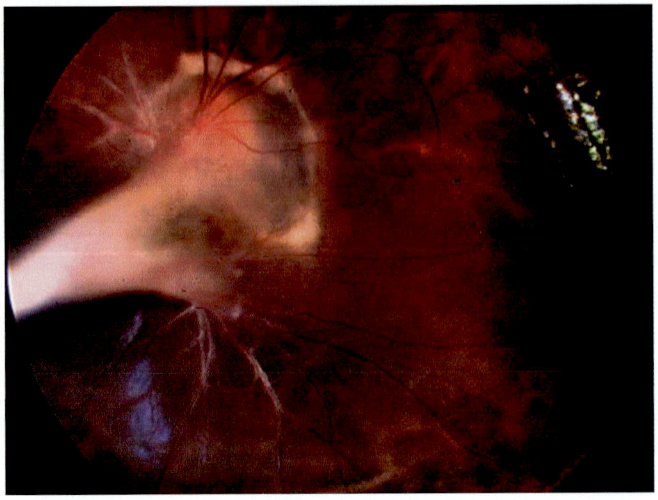

Fig. 6.2 Posterior PFV showing stalk extending from the optic disc with tractional retinal detachment

2. *Posterior PFV:* It has predominant features of persistent posterior hyaloid artery without much or any anterior tunica vasculosa lentis:
   (a) Microphthalmos (may or may not be present).
   (b) Posterior lens opacity.
   (c) Vitreous stalk. The stalk can insert anteriorly on the lens either centrally, involving the visual axis, or eccentrically (nasally), sparing the visual axis of the lens. If the stalk is eccentric (Fig. 6.2), no change in visual acuity is noticed in the very young child, but often presents with strabismus later in life, at age 9–10 months (Shaikh and Trese 2003). If there is visual axis opacity, the problem usually is discovered earlier.
   (d) Retinal fold with tractional retinal detachment (Fig. 6.3).
   (e) Retinal dysplasia, which can be divided into macroscopic and microscopic types (Trese and Capone Jr. 2014). Macroscopic dysplasia is defined as changes easily visible with the operating microscope/indirect ophthalmoscope; microscopic dysplasia occurs at the cellular or vascular level. Fluorescein angiography is helpful in these cases.
   (f) Hypoplastic optic nerve and macula.

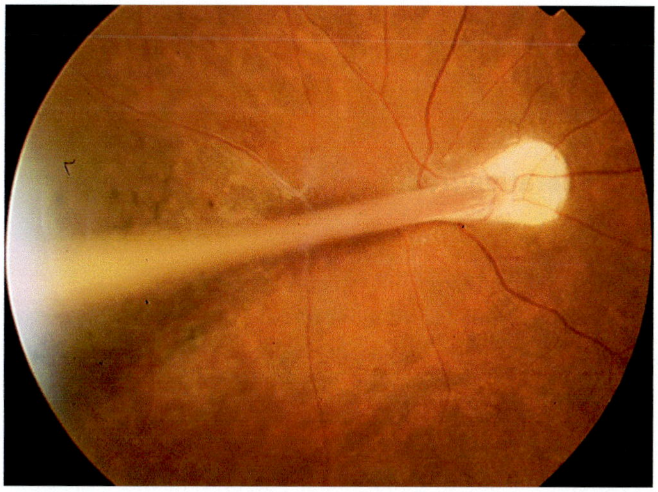

Fig. 6.3 Posterior PFV with nasal retinal fold

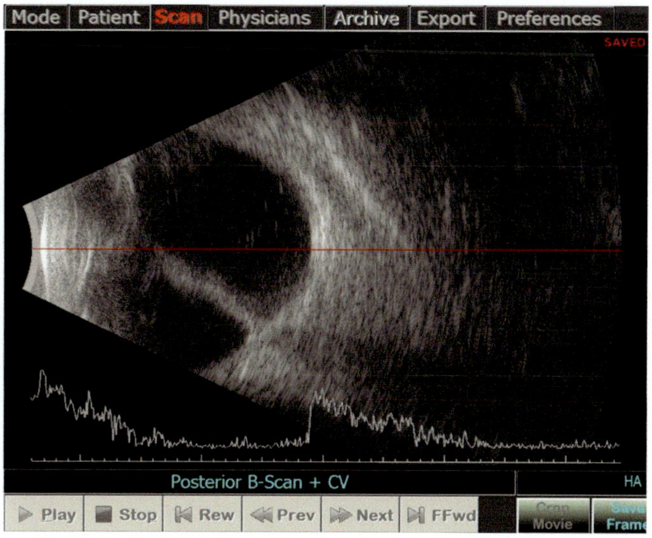

Fig. 6.4 B scan photo showing a thick band extending anteriorly from the optic nerve head

Posterior PFV is further divided into mild and severe involvement (Dass and Trese 1999). Mild cases included only elevated vitreous membrane with a stalk from the optic nerve. All other cases were considered as severe involvement.

3. *Mixed PFV:* Features of both anterior and posterior PFV.

Other ocular and systemic associations

PFV may be associated with central nervous system abnormalities (Marshman et al. 1999), tuberous sclerosis (Milot et al. 1999), oral–facial–digital syndrome (Tsai and O'Brien 1999), intrauterine herpes simplex infection (Corey and Flynn 2000), intrauterine exposure to clomiphene (Bishai et al. 1999), and MPPC (microcornea, posterior lenticonus, persistent fetal vasculature and coloboma) (Ranchod et al. 2010).

Investigations

1. B scan ultrasound (Byrne and Green 2002): Echography usually shows a shorter than normal globe, although it may be normal in some patients. The lens is often thin, and there may be irregularity of the posterior capsule. A retrolental membrane can sometimes be demonstrated. A vitreous band (persistent hyaloid vessel) may be seen extending from the posterior lens capsule to the optic disc. Very often this band is extremely thin and difficult to identify along its entire course. In other situations, it can be thick and easy to demonstrate (Fig. 6.4). Sometimes a tractional retinal detachment can be seen posteriorly which can help it differentiate from a closed funnel retinal detachment.

   B-scan is mandatory to rule out the differential diagnosis.
2. Ultrasound biomicroscopy (UBM): Can show the fibrous membrane behind the lens, mainly to rule out medulloepithelioma or other benign tumors of ciliary body which may have similar presentation. May require general anesthesia.
3. Fundus fluorescein angiography (FFA): To detect vascular dysplasia where capillary-free zone is seen and to prognosticate surgical outcome. To support the diagnosis of PFV by showing the brittle star pattern of vasculature in the fibrous tissue (Reese 1955).
4. Computed tomographic scanning and magnetic resonance imaging are rarely needed, mainly to rule out retinoblastoma in doubtful cases.
5. Visual evoked potential testing may be useful in predicting retinal dysplasia (Dass and Trese 1999). If a response is present, then it can be helpful in the decision whether to recommend surgery for retinal detachment. This is most helpful when the other eye is uninvolved, and the waveforms can be compared.

Management

PFV is a non-progressive disorder, although tractional intraocular changes can occur later, most likely due to eye growth. The stalk also can cause traction on the posterior lens capsule leading to posterior lenticonus. Traction on the ciliary body can lead to hypotony. Traction on the retina leads to tractional retinal detachment.

Observation

If there are subtle persistent fetal vasculature changes which do not affect the visual axis, then the child is only observed and refractive correction with amblyopia management advised. On the other side of the spectrum, if the eye is severely microphthalmic with a closed funnel retinal detachment with subretinal opacities, then these eyes also need to be only observed and proper cosmetic correction given.

Surgery

Anterior PFV: It is managed similar to congenital cataract where through scleral tunnel lens aspiration is done followed by primary posterior capsulotomy followed by removal of the fibrous membrane and anterior vitrectomy. Bleeders are managed by diathermy. Post-operatively refraction and aggressive amblyopia management is required. Posterior chamber intraocular lens (PCIOL) can be placed in children more than 6 months of age in sulcus if capsular rim can be kept intact. Anterior PFV is best managed by pediatric ophthalmologists as they can preserve the capsular rim for future secondary PCIOL implantation.

Posterior PFV: Surgery is not required if no traction is on lens capsule or retina and visual axis is clear. Lens-sparing vitrectomy (Dass and Trese 1999) is the surgery of choice (however, lensectomy is mostly needed due to the close proximity with the lens). Entry is through pars plicata (as pars plana is still not developed in infants). Thus, entry is 1–1.5 mm from limbus to avoid creation of iatrogenic breaks. After core vitrectomy the stalk is cut. Caution should be exercised before cutting the stalk as intrinsic retinal vessels can be present in it. If doubtful, stalk can be pushed from side to side before dividing to determine any retinal circulation alteration. If intrinsic vessels present, then the stalk is usually cut anteriorly. The surgeon should be aware of this as great care is required to divide only stalk tissue, not retina or intrinsic retinal vessels which could lead to a retinal hole or bleeding, followed by a retinal ischemic event. At the end, fluid air exchange can be done.

Mixed PFV: Cataract aspiration is done as anterior PFV. This is followed by three-port vitrectomy either through the limbal paracentesis using anterior chamber maintainer or through the pars plicata after making the ports 1 mm from limbus.

Care should be taken during surgical removal of fibrous membrane and peripheral vitrectomy as it can easily lead to iatrogenic retinal dialysis.

Postoperative Treatment

- Surgery alone does not constitute treatment.
- Aggressive management of amblyopia by way of contact lenses, aphakic glasses, or secondary PCIOL implantation is needed to have a good visual outcome.

Early surgical intervention followed by adequate amblyopic therapy leads to good visual outcome in these patients. Various studies show that the visual outcome in PFV cases post-surgery depends on the severity of posterior segment involvement and aggressive amblyopia therapy (Dass and Trese 1999; Scott et al. 1989; Federman et al. 1982; Alexandrakis et al. 2000; Mittra et al. 1998). We did a retrospective, non-comparative interventional study in our center from the period of 2006 to 2016. Fifteen eyes of 13 patients with PFV were analyzed. Two (15.4%) patients were diagnosed with bilateral PFV. Although distinction between bilateral PFV and Norrie disease was not defined by molecular genetic analysis, Norrie disease has more severe hemorrhagic and dysplastic retinal detachment (deJuan Jr et al. 2001), which was not seen in our cases. Twelve (92.3%) patients presented with leukocoria. Thirteen (83.3%) eyes had both anterior and posterior PFV. Two patients had associated disc coloboma and two patients had vitreous hemorrhage in association with PFV. Initial lensectomy was done in eight (53.3%) eyes, lensectomy with vitrectomy in five (33.3%) eyes, and lens-sparing vitrectomy in two eyes (13.3%). Final best corrected visual acuity ranged from fixing and following light to 6/18. In our study too, absence of severe posterior involvement was a predictor of better visual outcome.

Visual Prognosis

The severity of anterior segment appearance, globe size, severity of lens involvement retinal dysplasia, and postsurgical effective amblyopic therapy often determine the eye's visual result.

Differential Diagnosis

1 Retinoblastoma.
2 Norrie disease: When bilateral PFV syndrome is present.

3 Congenital cataract.
4 Familial exudative vitreoretinopathy.
5 Incontinentia pigmenti.
6 Stage 5 Retinopathy of prematurity.

Conclusion

- With modern vitreoretinal techniques, good visual results are possible. Smaller gauge 25 and even 27G instruments (Video 6.1) can be used for vitrectomy.
- However, good anatomical and visual outcome depends on
  - Timing of intervention
  - Anatomy of posterior pole
  - Amount of anisometropia
  - Amblyopia management

References

Alexandrakis G, Scott IU, Flynn HW Jr, Murray TG, Feuer WJ. Visual acuity outcomes with and without surgery in patients with persistent fetal vasculature. Ophthalmology. 2000;107:1068–72.

Azuma M, Yamaguchi Y, Handa H, Hayakawa M, Kanai A, Yamada M. Mutations of the PAX6 gene detected in patients with a variety of optic-nerve malformations. Am J Hum Genet. 2003;72:1565–70.

Bishai R, Arbour L, Lyons C, Koren G. Intrauterine exposure to clomiphene and neonatal persistent hyperplastic primary vitreous. Teratology. 1999;60:143–5.

Byrne SF, Green RL. Intraocular tumors. In: Byrne SF, Green RL, editors. Ultrasound of the eye and orbit. 2nd ed. St. Louis: Mosby; 2002. p. 115–90.

Corey RP, Flynn JT. Maternal intrauterine herpes simplex virus infection leading to persistent fetal vasculature. Arch Ophthalmol. 2000;118:837–40.

Dass AB, Trese MT. Persistent hyperplastic primary vitreous results. Ophthalmology. 1999;106:280–4.

deJuan E Jr, Farr A, Noorily S. Retinal detachment in infants. In: Ryan SJ, Wilkinson CP, editors. Retina, vol. 3. 3rd ed. St. Louis: Mosby; 2001. p. 2501.

Federman JL, Shields JA, Altman B, Koller B. The surgical and non surgical management of persistent hyperplastic primary vitreous. Ophthalmology. 1982;89:20–4.

Goldberg MF. Persistent fetal vasculature (PFV): an integrated interpretation of signs and symptoms associated with persistent hyperplastic primary vitreous (PHPV). LIV Edward Jackson Memorial Lecture. Am J Ophthalmol. 1997;124:587–626.

Khaliq S, Hameed A, Ismail M, Anwar K, Leroy B, Payne AM, et al. Locus for autosomal recessive nonsyndromic persistent hyperplastic primary vitreous. Invest Ophthalmol Vis Sci. 2001;42:2225–8.

Marshman WE, Jan JE, Lyons CJ. Neurologic abnormalities associated with persistent hyperplastic primary vitreous. Can J Ophthalmol. 1999;34:17–22.

Meeson A, Palmer M, Calfon M, et al. A relationship between apoptosis and flow during programmed capillary regression is revealed by vital analysis. Development. 1996;122:3929.

Milot J, Michaud J, Lemieux N, et al. Persistent hyperplastic primary vitreous with retinal tumor in tuberous sclerosis: report of a case including tumoral immunohistochemistry and cytogenetic analyses. Ophthalmology. 1999;106:630–4.

Mittra RA, Huynh LT, Ruttum MS, Mieler WF, Connor TB, Han DP, et al. Visual outcomes following lensectomy and vitrectomy for combined anterior and posterior persistent hyperplastic primary vitreous. Arch Ophthalmol. 1998;116:1190–4.

Ranchod TM, Quiram PA, Hathaway N, Ho LY, Glasgow BJ, Trese MT. Microcornea, posterior megalolenticonus, persistent fetal vasculature, and coloboma: a new syndrome. Ophthalmology. 2010;117:1843–7.

Reese AB. Persistent hyperplastic primary vitreous. Am J Ophthalmo.l. 1955;40:317–31.

Scott WE, Drummond GT, Keech RV, Karr DJ. Management and visual acuity results of monocular congenital cataracts and persistent hyperplastic primary vitreous. Aust N Z J Ophthalmol. 1989;17:143–51.

Sebag J. Vitreous structure. In: Albert DM, Jakobiec FA, editors. Principles and practice of ophthalmology, vol. 3. Philadelphia, PA: W. B. Saunders Company; 2000. p. 1792–3.

Sebag J, Nguven N. Embryology of the posterior segment and developmental disorders. B. Vitreous embryology and vitreo-retinal developmental disorders. In: Hartnett ME, editor. Pediatric retina. Philadelphia: Lippincott Williams & Wilkins; 2005. p. 13–28.

Shaikh S, Trese MT. Lens-sparing vitrectomy in predominantly posterior persistent fetal vasculature syndrome in eyes with nonaxial lens opacification. Retina. 2003;23:330–4.

Trese MT, Capone A Jr. Diagnosis and management of persistent fetal vasculature syndrome. In: Hartnett ME, editor. Pediatric retina. 2nd ed. Philadelphia: Lippincott Williams & Wilkins; 2014. p. 626–32.

Tsai PS, O'Brien JM. Retinal hamartoma in oral-facial-digital syndrome. Arch Ophthalmol. 1999;117:963–5.

Familial Exudative Vitreoretinopathy

7

Julia Shulman, Jonathan Feistmann,
and M. Elizabeth Hartnett

Introduction

Familial exudative vitreoretinopathy (FEVR) is a clinically heterogeneous disorder of retinal vascular development characterized by peripheral retinal ischemia that can lead to retinal neovascularization, dragging of the retinal vessels, fold formation, hyaloid contraction, and tractional retinal detachments (Kashani et al. 2014).

It was first described by Criswick and Schepens (1969). In 1976, Canny and Oliver described the peripheral vascular abnormalities and non-perfusion characteristics of FEVR (Canny and Oliver 1976). The modern classification of FEVR describes five stages and incorporates both clinical and angiographic findings of the disease (Table 7.1) (Kashani et al. 2014).

The patterns of inheritance and expressivity in FEVR are heterogeneous with several genes implicated in the pathogenesis.

The use of wide-field angiography has ushered in an era of better understanding and classification of the peripheral vascular abnormalities as well as identification of peripheral avascular retina, in early asymptomatic cases or in minimally affected family members. In addition, the availability of wide-field angiography in infants has improved our ability to distinguish FEVR from ROP in preterm infants (John et al. 2016).

The disease can be progressive in childhood and adolescence. Younger patients diagnosed with FEVR have a poorer visual prognosis when compared with adults (Gilmour 2015). FEVR is a lifelong disease that can range from being stable and asymptomatic to being vision threatening and progressive resulting in poor visual outcomes despite treatment (Sizmaz et al. 2015).

Table 7.1 Clinical classification of FEVR

Stage	Description
1A	Avascular peripheral retina or anomalous intraretinal vascularization, *without* extraretinal vascularization, *without* exudate or leakage
1B	Avascular peripheral retina or anomalous intraretinal vascularization, *without* extraretinal vascularization *with* exudate or leakage
2A	Avascular peripheral retina *with* extraretinal vascularization, *without* exudate or leakage
2B	Avascular peripheral retina *with* extraretinal vascularization, *with* exudate or leakage
3A	Extramacular retinal detachment *without* exudate or leakage
3B	Extramacular retinal detachment *with* exudate or leakage
4A	Macula-involving retinal detachment *without* exudate or leakage
4B	Macula-involving retinal detachment *with* exudate or leakage
5A	Total retinal detachment—open funnel
5B	Total retinal detachment—closed funnel

Based on classification by Pendergast and Trese (1998), updated in 2014 (Kashani et al. 2014)

Pathogenesis

A positive family history is found in 20–40% of FEVR cases. The inheritance of FEVR can be autosomal dominant, recessive, and X-linked recessive, with the autosomal dominant form being most common; the remainder of cases are novel mutations (Ranchod et al. 2011). At the time of this writing, six genes have been identified in the pathogenesis of FEVR—*NDP, FZD4, LRP5, TSPAN12, ZNF408,* and *KIF11*. Mutations in these genes account for 50% of FEVR cases, and four of the protein products of these genes play a role in the Wnt signaling pathway that is critical in retinal angiogenesis (Gilmour 2015; Sizmaz et al. 2015; Robitaille et al. 2014). Table 7.2 summarizes the known genes, chromosomal

J. Shulman
New York Medical College, Turo, Valhalla, NY, USA

New York Eye and Ear Infirmary of Mount Sinai,
New York, NY, USA

J. Feistmann
New York Eye and Ear Infirmary of Mount Sinai,
New York, NY, USA

M. E. Hartnett (✉)
Moran Eye Center, University of Utah, Salt Lake City, UT, USA
e-mail: me.hartnett@hsc.utah.edu

R. V. P. Chan (ed.), *Pediatric Retinal Diseases*, Retina Atlas, https://doi.org/10.1007/978-981-19-1364-8_7

location, and disease phenotype known to be caused by the gene.

Knockout mouse models of four of the known FEVR genes show the absence of the deeper retinal plexuses in the presence of a formed primary retinal plexus; however, this has not been demonstrated clinically in humans (Xia et al. 2008; Xu et al. 2004; Richter et al. 1998). It is postulated that FEVR is a disorder of angiogenesis in which the primary vascular plexus develops normally, but the capillary layers in the deep and peripheral retina are abnormal (Gilmour 2015).

In cases where FEVR clinically progresses, the avascular peripheral retina leads to intravitreous neovascularization which leads to subsequent complications including vitreoretinal traction and tractional retinal detachment, macular dragging, and retinal folds (Image 7.1—macular dragging and fold). Additionally, progression of FEVR can lead to exudative changes with serous retinal detachment.

Table 7.2 Genes implicated in FEVR

Gene	Protein product	Chromosome	Diseases caused
NDP	Norrin Disease Protein	X-chromosome	X-linked recessive FEVR, Norrie Disease
FZD4	Frizzled-4	Chromosome 11	AD FEVR
LRP5	Low-density lipoprotein receptor-related protein 5	Chromosome 11	AD and AR FEVR
TSPAN12	Tetraspanin-12	Chromosome 7	AD FEVR
ZNF408	Zinc finger protein 408	Chromosome 11	AD FEVR
KIF11	Kinesin like protein family 11	Chromosome 10	AD FEVR, can be associated with microcephaly

AD autosomal dominant, *AR* autosomal recessive

Though FEVR was classically described in full-term infants, there are pre-term infants who exhibit a course and fluorescein angiographic findings consistent with FEVR, giving rise to a new classification of ROPER (ROP vs. FEVR) (John et al. 2016). These patients have bulbous vascular terminals, capillary dropout, venous–venous shunting, and abnormal branching patterns on angiography (Image 7.2—ROPER). Unlike ROP, ROPER can re-activate after an episode of quiescence, similar to FEVR. These patients need to follow up with periodic exams and wide-field angiography (John et al. 2016).

Clinical Features

FEVR has a variable presentation within the same family with the same gene variant or even within the same patient. The disease course can also vary with some patients having progressive loss of capillaries and capillary non-perfusion but others having stable retinal exams for extended periods of time.

The most common and unifying clinical finding in FEVR is avascular peripheral retina, which may be present in one or both eyes (Image 7.3). Other findings include macular dragging, retinal folds, neovascularization at the vascular avascular junction (Image 7.4), vitreoretinal proliferation and traction, as well as subretinal exudation. Retinal vessels can demonstrate excessive branching with bifurcations having more right angles in the periphery and more vessels radiating from the optic disc in the posterior pole (Miner et al. 2017). In addition to the peripheral vascular non-perfusion, there can be areas of capillary dropout within the vascularized retina.

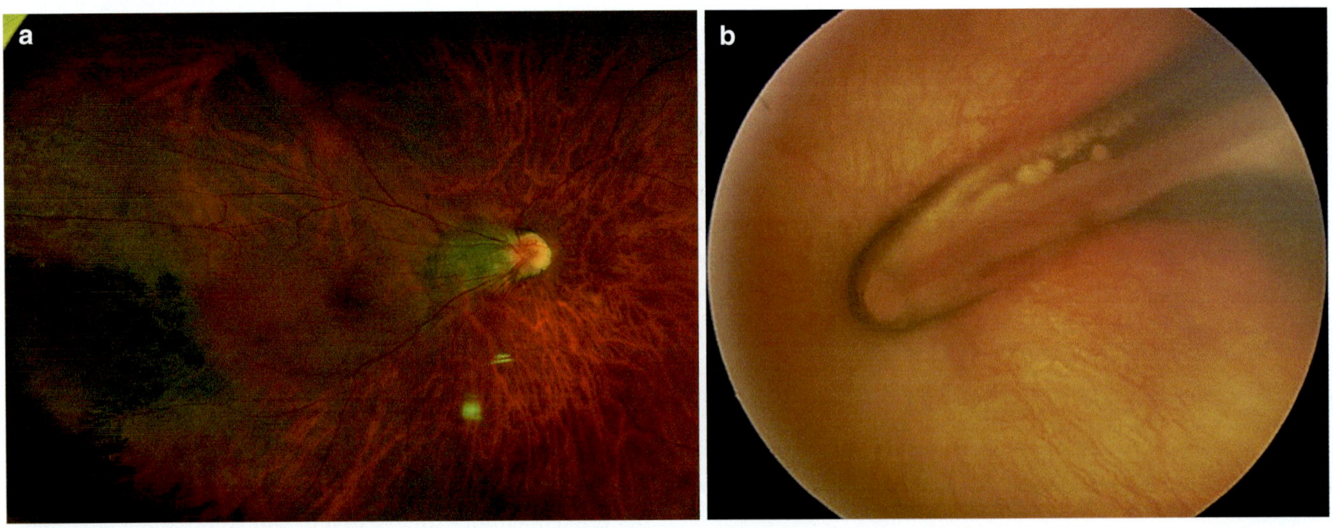

Image 7.1 (**a**) Macular dragging and peripheral pigmentary changes. (**b**) Macular falciform fold

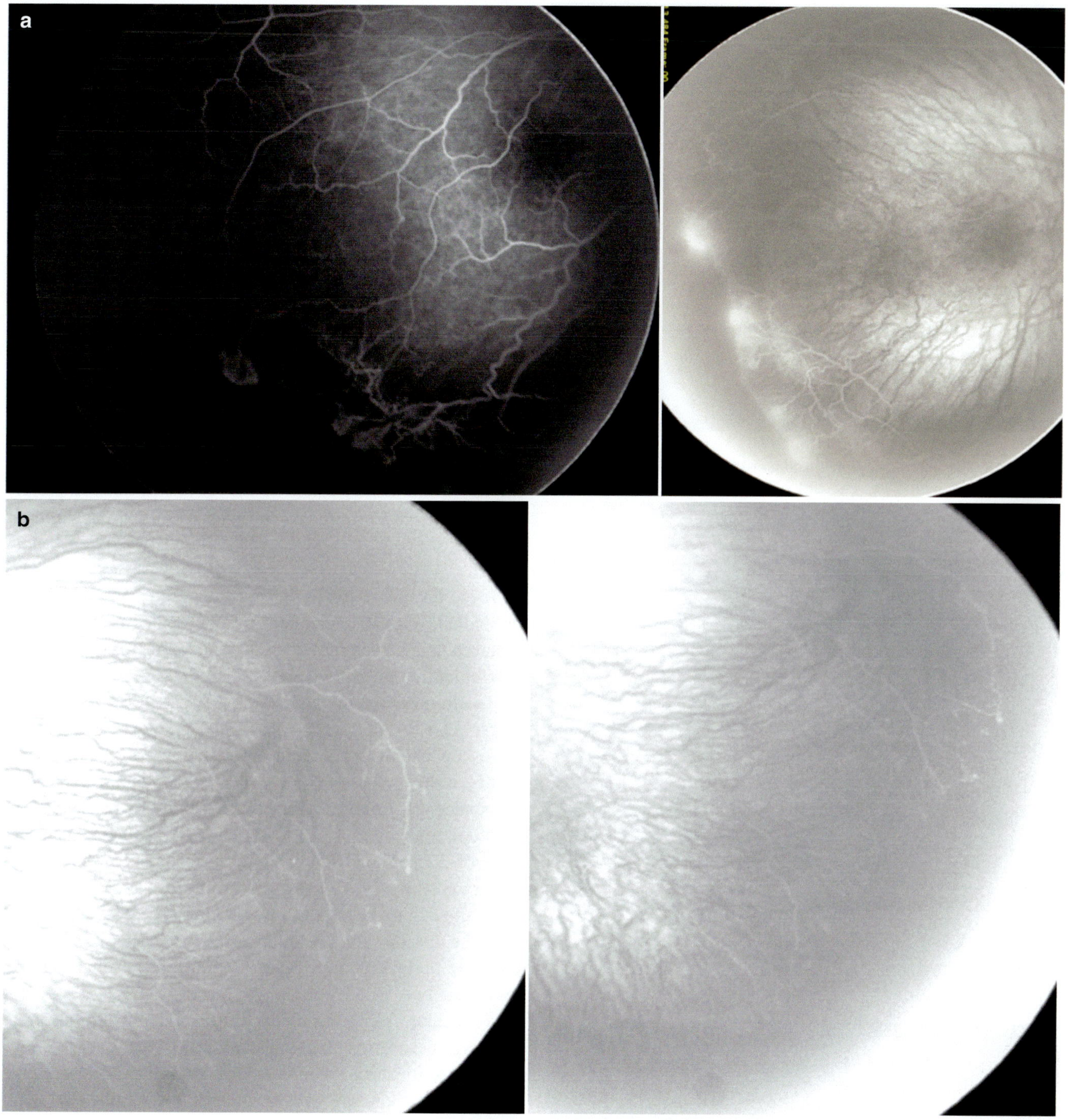

Image 7.2 ROP versus FEVR. 26 weeks' gestational age twin, FA done at 60 weeks' PMA (postmenstrual age) demonstrating (**a**) bulb-like aneurysmal dilatations, capillary dropout, and abnormal leakage and (**b**) aneurysmal dilatations of the vessels

In more severe cases, there can be severe macular dragging, folds, and retinal detachment (tractional or combined tractional/rhegmatogenous) (Image 7.5—FEVR detachment).

A careful examination of the patient and family members as well as wide-field fluorescein angiography is essential in making the diagnosis. Classic angiography findings include vascular dilation at the vascular–avascular junction, vascular loops, and bulb-like telangiectatic endings with focal or massive areas of leakage (Image 7.6—peripheral FA of FEVR).

Spectral domain OCT has shown posterior hyaloid organization, vitreomacular traction, diminished foveal contour, persistent fetal foveal architecture, cystoid macular edema, intraretinal exudates and subretinal lipid aggregation, dry or

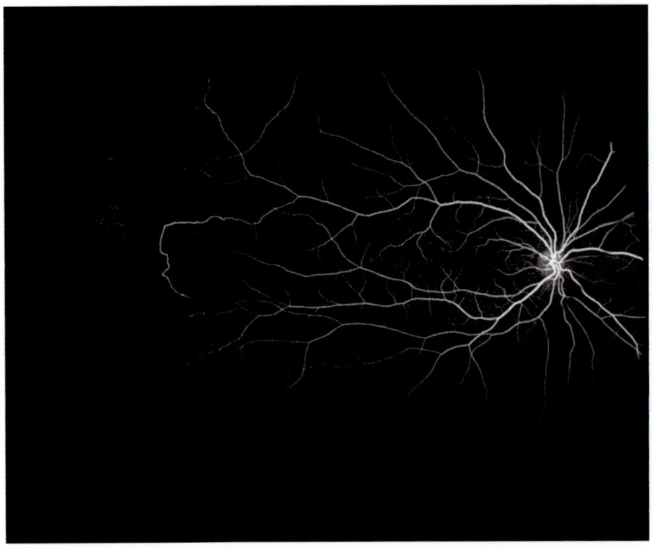

Image 7.3 Fluorescein angiogram demonstrating peripheral avascular retina, circumferential vessels, and bulb-like aneurysmal dilatations (Stage 1A)

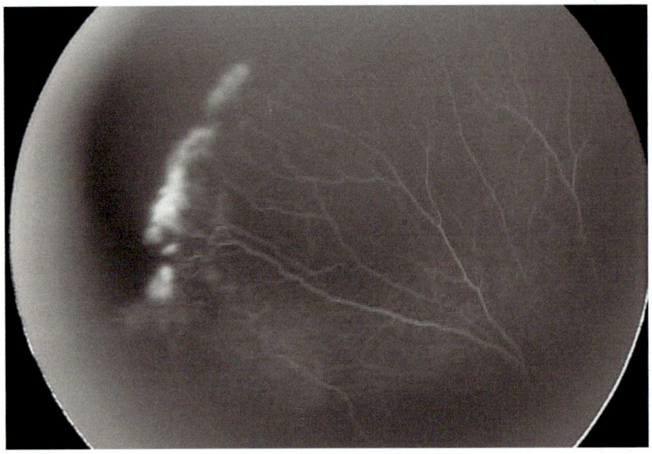

Image 7.4 Neovascularization at the vascular–avascular junction on FA (Stage 2A)

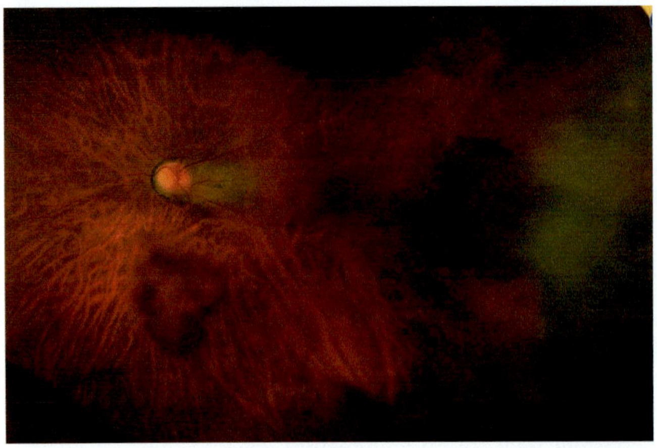

Image 7.5 Macular dragging, pigmentary changes, and peripheral FEVR detachment

edematous radial folds, and disruption of the ellipsoid zone (Image 7.7—OCT in FEVR) (Yonekawa et al. 2015).

Management

The hallmark of treatment for FEVR is laser photocoagulation to the avascular retina. Stage 1 FEVR may not require treatment and requires regular follow-up with periodic fluorescein angiography. Even in advanced cases that involve detachment of the retina, laser to the peripheral avascular retina can result in an improved anatomic outcome.

Although regression of neovascularization with good anatomic outcome has been described in adult FEVR treated with intravitreal bevacizumab (IVB) (Tagami et al. 2008) and IVB has been used in conjunction with laser ablation or surgery to repair a retinal detachment in pediatric patients, the role of anti-vascular endothelial growth factor (VEGF) therapy in the management of FEVR is still not completely clear. It has been reported that tractional retinal detachments can progress after use of intravitreal anti-VEGF (Henry et al. 2015).

If the disease is treated promptly, progression to RD can be halted. FEVR-associated retinal detachments can be repaired using a scleral buckle (SB) or vitrectomy (PPV), or a combination of the two.

Tractional retinal detachments associated with stage 3 or worse FEVR can present a surgical challenge. In a large series on anatomic outcomes in pediatric retinal detachments, a 40% anatomic success was reported with FEVR-associated tractional retinal detachments (10 patients were included in the analysis) (Read et al. 2018). In a series of 31 eyes of 22 patients (age range 1 month to 18 years) who underwent surgery, 12 eyes underwent SB, 1 SB and PPV, 7 PPV alone, and 11 lensectomy and PPV. 26 eyes reattached after the first surgery. The authors advocate scleral buckles in cases of peripheral fibrovascular proliferation that extends less than two clock hours. For more extensive peripheral fibrovascular proliferation or traction on the posterior retina, PPV was performed (Yamane et al. 2014). Similar outcomes were described in a single-center study of 34 years that underwent vitrectomy with or without lensectomy (Fei et al. 2016).

Medical Considerations

Greater understanding of the early findings of FEVR has been obtained with wide-angle and ultra-wide-field FA and through genetic testing and evaluation of family members of patients with clinical manifestations of FEVR. Experimental studies have opened doors to potential medical management to prevent late complications and vision loss in FEVR. As mentioned earlier, agents that inhibit the bioactivity of vas-

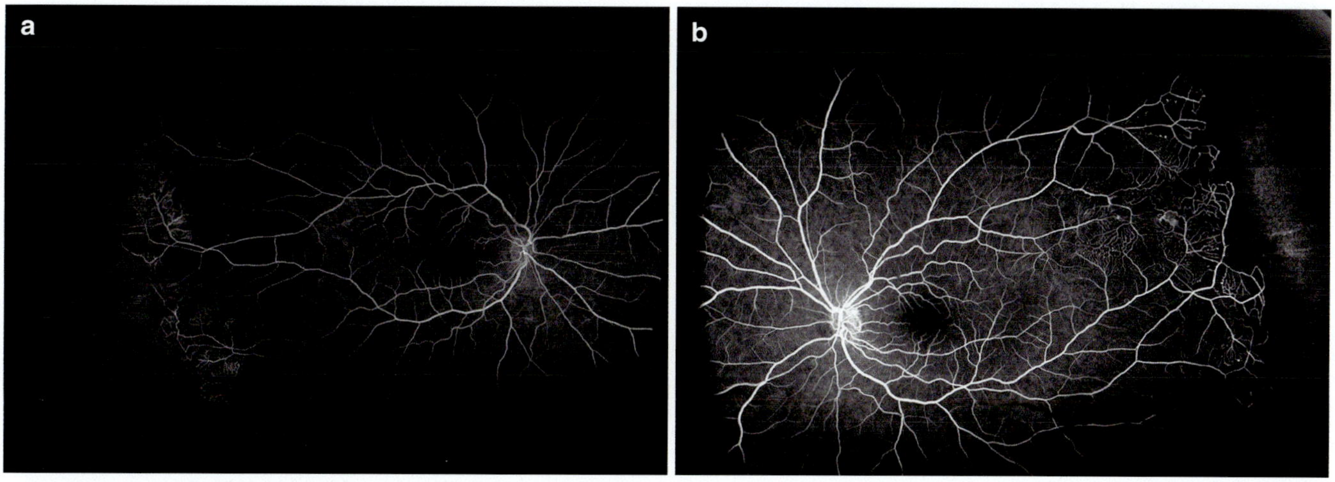

Image 7.6 (**a**) Peripheral avascular retina and capillary dropout. (**b**) Bulb-like aneurysmal dilations, capillary dropout (Stage 1B)

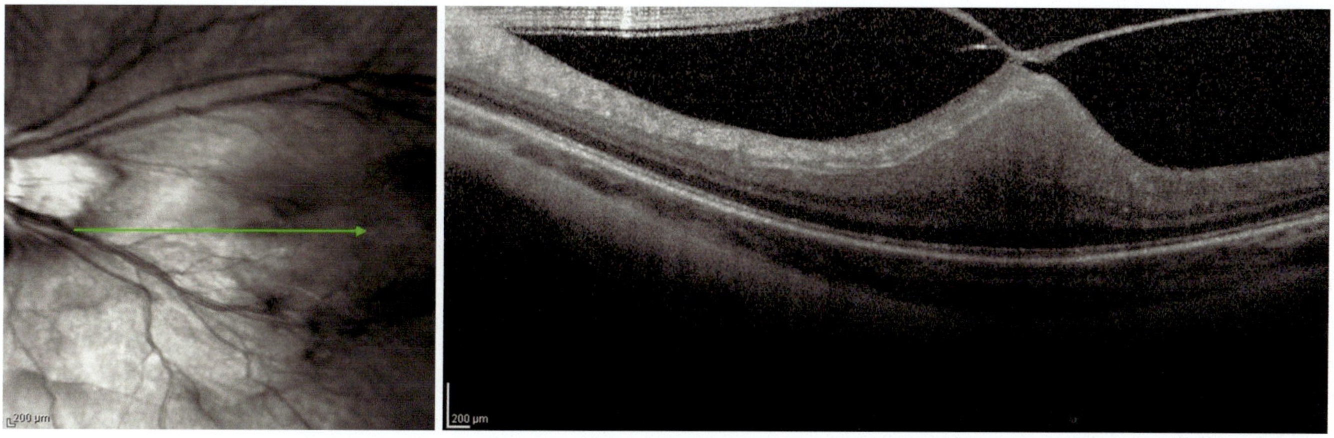

Image 7.7 OCT in FEVR demonstrating vitreous organization and traction in the macula in a patient with significant macular fold

cular endothelial growth factor (VEGF) are anti-angiogenic and reduce permeability of vessels. However, it is becoming increasingly recognized that some patients with FEVR have progressive capillary dropout at certain stages in their lives.

Capillary dropout related to endothelial cell dysfunction underlies other conditions including Coats' disease and diabetic retinopathy and many times may be preceded by the presence of staining of the retinal capillaries. Wide-field fluorescein angiography is valuable to identify capillary dropout and staining of capillaries, described as late-phase angiographic posterior and peripheral vascular leakage (Thanos et al. 2016). In experimental models of retinopathy, the use of Norrin was found to rescue vasculature in mice by improved endothelial barrier integrity (Tokunaga et al. 2013). Norrin is a ligand that binds the coreceptors, LRP5 and FZD4, in the Wnt signaling pathway. More studies are indicated to understand potential mechanisms for progression of FEVR and opportunities for intervention to treat it.

References

Canny CL, Oliver GL. Fluorescein angiographic findings in familial exudative vitreoretinopathy. Arch Ophthalmol. 1976;94:1114–20.

Criswick VG, Schepens CL. Familial exudative vitreoretinopathy. Am J Ophthalmol. 1969;68:578–94.

Fei P, Yang W, Zhang Q. Surgical management of advanced familial exudative vitreoretinopathy with complications. Retina. 2016;36(8):1480–5.

Gilmour DF. Familial exudative vitreoretinopathy and related retinopathies. Eye. 2015;29:1–14.

Henry CR, Sisk RA, Tzu JH, et al. Long-term follow-up of intravitreal bevacizumab for the treatment of pediatric retinal and choroidal diseases. J AAPOS. 2015;19(6):541–8.

John VJ, McClintic JI, Hess JD, et al. Retinopathy of prematurity versus familial exudative vitreoretinopathy: report on clinical and angiographic findings. Ophthal Surg Lasers Imaging Retina. 2016;47:14–9.

Kashani AH, Brown KT, Chang E, et al. Diversity of retinal vascular anomalies in patients with familial exudative vitreoretinopathy. Ophthalmology. 2014;121:2220–7.

Miner Y, Yang Y, Yan H, et al. Increased posterior retinal vessels in mild asymptomatic familial exudative vitreoretinopathy eyes. Retina. 2017;36(6):1209–15.

Pendergast SD, Trese MT. Familial exudative vitreoretinopathy. Results of surgical management. Ophthalmology. 1998;105(6):1015–23.

Ranchod MT, Ho LY, Drenser KA, et al. Clinical presentation of familial exudative vitreoretinopathy. Ophthlamology. 2011;121:262–8.

Read SP, Aziz HA, Kuriyan A. Retina. 2018;August

Richter M, Gottanka J, May CA, et al. Retinal vascular changes in Norrie Disease mice. Invest Ophthalmol Vis Sci. 1998;39:2450–7.

Robitaille JM, Gillett RM, LeBlanc MA, et al. Phenotypic overlap between familial exudative vitreoretinopathy and microcephaly, lymphedema, and chorioretinal dysplasia caused by KIF11 mutations. JAMA Ophthalmol. 2014;132:1393–9.

Sizmaz S, Yonekawa Y, Trese MT. Familial exudative vitreoretinopathy. Turk J Ophthalmol. 2015;45:164–8.

Tagami M, Kusuhara S, Honda S. Rapid regression of retinal hemorrhage and neovascularization in a case of familial exudative vitreoretinopathy treated with intravitreal bevacizumab. Graefes Arch Clin Exp Ophthalmol. 2008;246(12):1787–9.

Thanos A, Bozho T, Trese M. A novel approach to understanding pathogenesis and treatment of capillary dropout in retinal vascular diseases. Ophthal Surg Lasers Imaging Retina. 2016;47(3):288–92.

Tokunaga CC, Chen YH, Dailey W, et al. A novel approach to understanding pathogenesis and treatment of capillary dropout in retinal vascular disease. Invest Ophthalmol Vis Sci. 2013;54(1):222–9.

Xia C, Liu H, Cheung D, et al. A model for familial exudative vitreoretinopathy caused by LPR5 mutations. Hum Mol Genet. 2008;17:1605–12.

Xu Q, Wang Y, Dabdoub A, et al. Vascular development in the retina and inner control by Norrin and Frizzled-4, a high affinity ligand receptor pair. Cell. 2004;116:883–95.

Yamane T, Tadashi Y, Nakayama Y, et al. Surgical outcomes of progressive tractional retinal detachment associated with familial exudative vitreoretinopathy. AJO. 2014;158(5):1049–55.

Yonekawa Y, Thomas BJ, Drenser KA, et al. Familial exudative vitreoretinopathy. Ophthalmology. 2015;122:2270–7.

8 Coats' Disease

Karen W. Jeng-Miller, Shizuo Mukai, and Yoshihiro Yonekawa

Introduction

Coats' disease is an idiopathic, non-hereditary retinal vascular disease. It was first described by George Coats in the early 1900s as a retinal vascular abnormality with retinal exudation occurring unilaterally in young men (Coats 1908). In 1912, Theodor Leber described a similar clinical entity of a retinal degeneration consisting of many miliary aneurysms with little to no exudation (Leber 1912). Subsequently in 1956, Aldernon Reese connected the two described entities and proposed that Leber's described miliary aneurysms were a precursor to the progressive retinal exudation described by Coats, and termed this spectrum of disease Coats' disease (Reese 1956).

Coats' disease most commonly affects young, healthy, males, although women can certainly be affected. It can present at any age, but the majority of patients are diagnosed within the first two decades of life (Char 2000; Egerer et al. 1974; Gomez 1965; Ridley et al. 1982; Tarkkanen and Laatikainen 1983). It is generally a unilateral condition, with 95% of cases being such; cases of bilateral involvement usually appear asymmetric, with minimal changes in the fellow eye (Shields et al. 2001a). There are no known systemic associations with the ocular findings of Coats' (Shields et al. 2001a). As a result, this disease should not be confused with other systemic diseases that present with bilateral Coats'-like exudative retinopathies, such as Coats' Plus disease, an autosomal recessive disorder resulting from mutations in the gene *conserved telomere maintenance component 1* (*CTC1*), which has similar ocular findings but systemic associations including dysplastic nails, intracranial calcifications, and sparse hair (Yannuzzi et al. 2014; Anderson et al. 2012; Tolmie et al. 1988). Patients with muscular dystrophies such as facioscapulohumeral muscular dystrophy (FSHD) may also present with bilateral Coats'-like exudative retinopathy (Vance et al. 2011; Statland et al. 2013; Ganesh et al. 2012). Therefore, a systemic workup should be considered if a child presents with relatively symmetric bilateral exudative retinopathies.

Classically, Coats' disease is characterized by unilateral retinal vascular telangiectasias and "light bulb" aneurysmal dilatations (Fig. 8.1), resulting in retinal exudation (Fig. 8.2) and exudative retinal detachment (Fig. 8.3) (Egerer et al. 1974; Tarkkanen and Laatikainen 1983; Shields et al. 2001a, b).

Clinical Features of Coats' Disease

Coats' disease has specific hallmark features used in clinical diagnosis. However, patients most often present with decreased vision, leukocoria, and/or strabismus, necessitating ruling out of life-threatening ocular conditions, most important being retinoblastoma (Shields et al. 2001a).

The classic telangiectasias and "light bulb" aneurysms of Coats' disease are most often found in the peripheral retina, most commonly in the temporal quadrant, but can extend posterior to the equator toward the vascular arcades and in all other quadrants also (Shields et al. 2001b; Shields and Shields 2002). However, it is rare to have telangiectasias in the macula, which occurs in less than 5% of cases (Shields and Shields 2002). Visual decline is usually precipitated by subretinal exudation. These exudates appear as yellow lipoproteinaceous deposits with diffuse retinal involvement and a particular affinity for the macula (Char 2000; Gomez 1965; Tarkkanen and Laatikainen 1983; Shields et al. 2001a). The

K. W. Jeng-Miller
Department of Ophthalmology and Visual Sciences, University of Massachusetts Medical School, Worcester, MA, USA

S. Mukai
Retina Service, Department of Ophthalmology, Massachusetts Eye and Ear Infirmary, Harvard Medical School, Boston, MA, USA

Y. Yonekawa (✉)
Retina Service, Wills Eye Hospital/Mid Atlantic Retina, Sidney Kimmel Medical College of Thomas Jefferson University, Philadelphia, PA, USA
e-mail: yyonekawa@midatlanticretina.com

R. V. P. Chan (ed.), *Pediatric Retinal Diseases*, Retina Atlas, https://doi.org/10.1007/978-981-19-1364-8_8

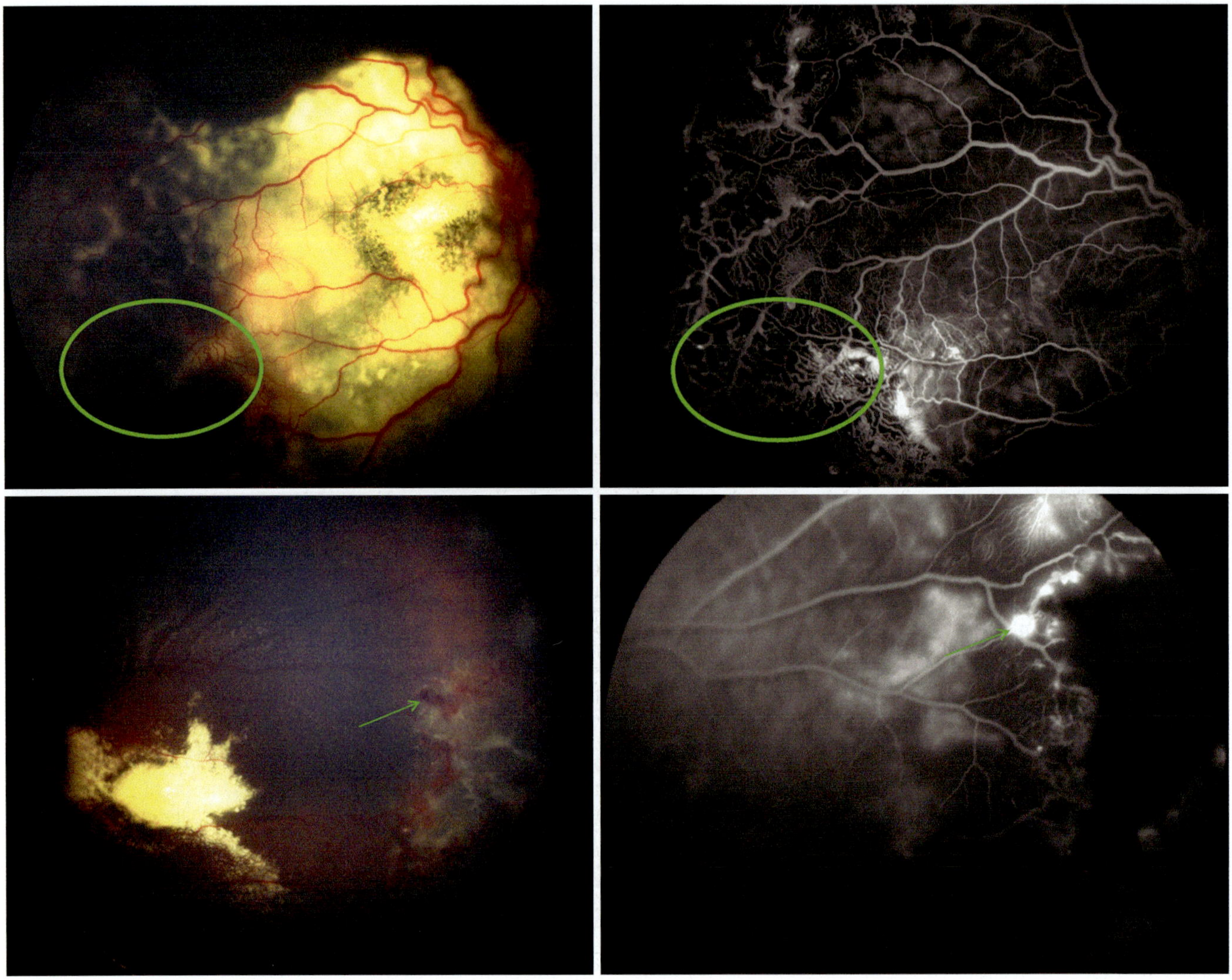

Fig. 8.1 Vascular telangiectasias (circle) and "light bulb" aneurysms (arrows) evident on wide-field fundus imaging (top) and fluorescein angiography (bottom) in Coats' disease

exudates have a propensity to accumulate in the macula despite the paucity of telangiectatic vessels in this area, because the peripheral exudates track posteriorly over time. Unfortunately, subfoveal exudate often results in a subfoveal nodule and evolve into macular fibrosis (Fig. 8.4), which portends a poorer visual prognosis (Shields et al. 2001b; Jumper et al. 2010; Khurana et al. 2005; Daruich et al. 2017). The subfoveal nodule is described as a yellow, exudative, protruding spheroidal lesion that can occur in as many as 52% of Coats' patients (Daruich et al. 2017). In cases of longitudinally observed subfoveal nodules, there is a 100% progression to macular fibrosis; in contrast, cases with subfoveal exudation without nodules progress to macular fibrosis approximately 15% of the time (Daruich et al. 2017).

When left untreated, Coats' disease unfortunately can progress to many advanced complications, such as exudative retinal detachments and secondary neovascular glaucoma, which can be especially devastating for vision (Tarkkanen and Laatikainen 1983; Shields et al. 2001a; Jumper et al. 2010; Khurana et al. 2005; Daruich et al. 2017; Ong et al. 2017). As a result, visual prognosis in Coats' disease is variable. Most patients (>50%) present with hand motion or worse vision (Shields et al. 2001a; Budning et al. 1998). The most important feature at the time of diagnosis to predict visual outcome of an eye with Coats' is the degree of peripheral retina that is involved with telangiectasias and the presence or absence of a retinal detachment; generally, those with improved visual acuity exhibited five or fewer clock hours of retinal telangiectasias without retinal detachment (Budning et al. 1998). Over the years, with advances in treatment methods and improved vision screenings at school and in the general pediatric office, children with Coats' disease have presented at an earlier stage, thereby undergoing earlier

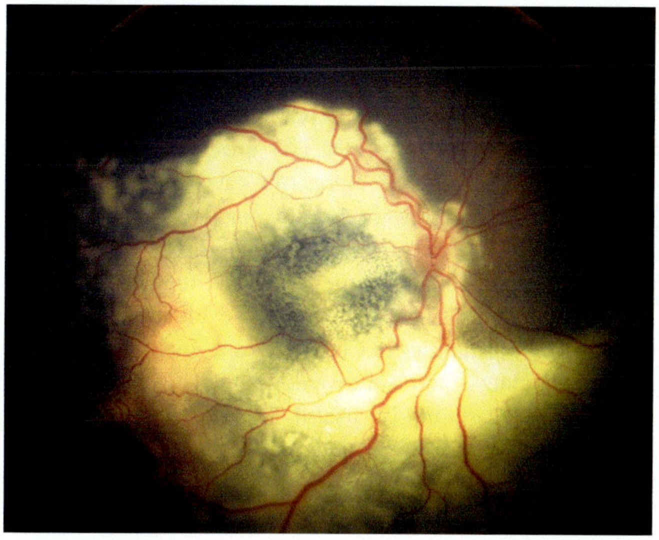

Fig. 8.2 Extensive exudates in the macula in Coats' disease

interventions and resulting in improved final visual outcomes (Ong et al. 2017).

Widefield Fundus Imaging and Fluorescein Angiography

Fluorescein angiography is the gold standard in the diagnosis of Coats' disease. There are many defining angiographic features, including the presence of peripheral nonperfusion, evidence of telangiectatic capillaries and "light bulb" aneurysms, and vascular leakage. Many of the pathologic vessels that result in visually significant changes are located in the periphery making them challenging to evaluate, especially in a pediatric population. Fortunately, new developments in imaging modalities, specifically wide-field fundus imaging and fluorescein angiography (WFA), have increased the ease of retinal examinations and become critical in the surveillance, diagnosis, and treatment of Coats' disease (Kang et al. 2013).

Wide-field fundus imaging provides a noninvasive snapshot of a significant portion of the retinal periphery. This is particularly useful in a pediatric population for which a reliable exam may not be easily accomplished. More importantly, WFA provides significantly more angiographic information regarding the retinal periphery and allows for better visualization of peripheral retinal vascular leakage and areas of non-perfusion. As a result, physicians can decrease the need to perform fluorescein angiography under anesthesia in the operating room in a predominately pediatric population, thus increasing the ease of obtaining serial fluorescein exams to monitor responses to treatment and development of new pathologies.

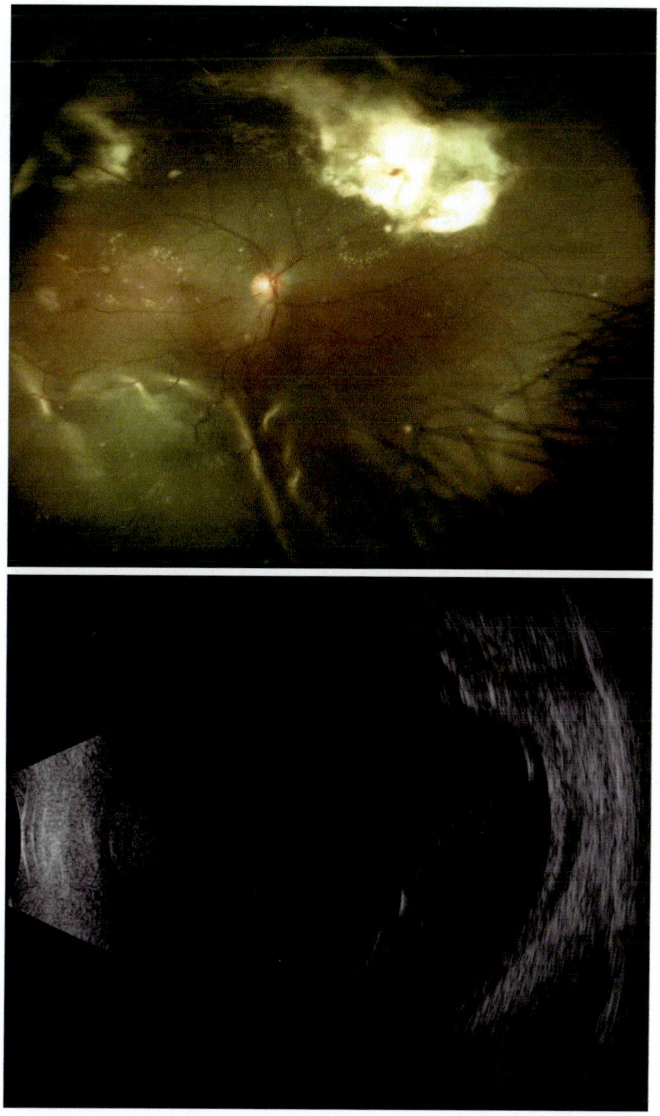

Fig. 8.3 Inferior exudative retinal detachment evident on wide-field fundus imaging (top) and B-scan ultrasonography (bottom)

The preferred method of obtaining WFA is intravenous fluorescein for outpatient WFA (such as with Optos California or Optos Tx, Optos, Marlborough, MA) in children who can tolerate intravenous access. This tends to be in older children, but may not be always possible. For younger children who can cooperate for fundus imaging but not intravenous access, oral fluorescein angiography can be performed. Only late-phase images are obtainable, and the signal strength may be limited. However, this is in general preferred over examinations under anesthesia (EUA), which we reserve for the youngest and least tolerant children. During EUAs, we perform contact camera WFA (such as with RetCam, Natus, Pleasantville, CA). Several other new cameras are now available also, such as the ICON camera (Phoenix Clinical, Pleasanton, CA) and PanoCam (Visunex, Fremont, CA).

Wide-field fluorescein angiogram has also been integral in studying and elucidating new pathologic findings in Coats' disease. While classically, known as a unilateral disease, recent studies have documented the existence of peripheral vascular and foveal changes in the unaffected (fellow) eye of patients with Coats' disease (Blair et al. 2013; Shane et al. 2011; Muakkassa et al. 2016; Jeng-Miller et al. 2017). In preliminary longitudinal studies, these lesions (Fig. 8.5) remain stable and do not progress or require treatment (Jeng-Miller et al. 2017).

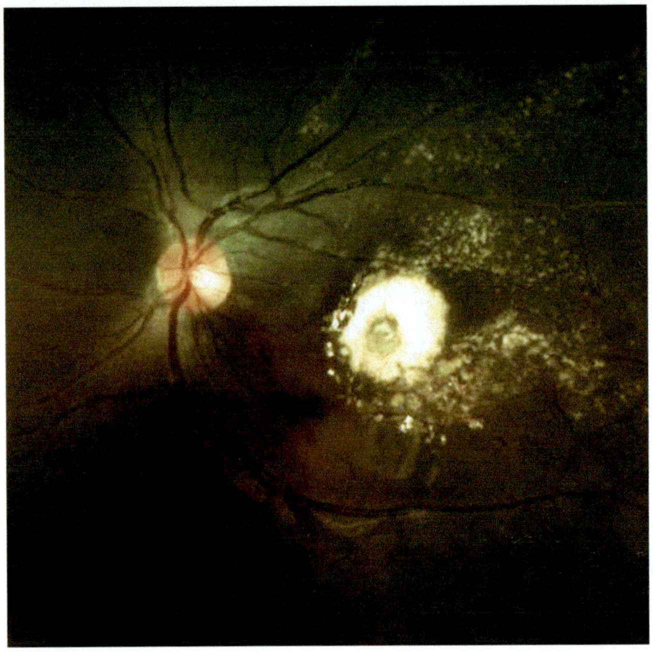

Fig. 8.4 Fundus photograph showing macular fibrosis and chronic exudates

Optical Coherence Tomography and Angiography

Optical coherence tomography (OCT) and optical coherence tomography angiography (OCTA) are increasingly being used to study pathologic features of Coats' disease as well as to longitudinally follow important macular exam findings. OCT and OCTA are noninvasive imaging modalities that require short examination times and defer the need for intravenous dye. OCT allows for precise evaluation of microstructural abnormalities in Coats' disease, including macular edema, exudates, and subfoveal nodules (Fig. 8.6). As a result, it is particularly useful for monitoring macular changes in response to treatment (Fig. 8.7). However, OCT only has the ability to evaluate the superficial and deep retinal layers of the macula, but it is not able to assess retinal microvasculature, a key aspect of Coats' pathology.

OCTA images the vascular plexuses at various retinal depths, in contrast to fluorescein angiography, which cannot

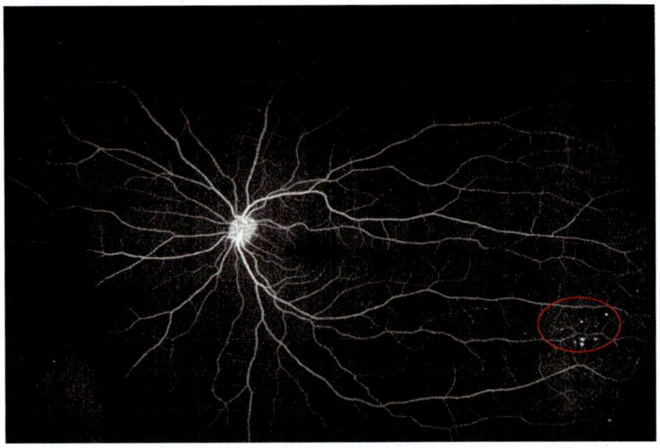

Fig. 8.5 Wide-field fluorescein angiography of a fellow eye in a patient with Coats' disease showing aneurysms (circle)

Fig. 8.6 Spectral domain optical coherence tomography demonstrating a subfoveal nodule

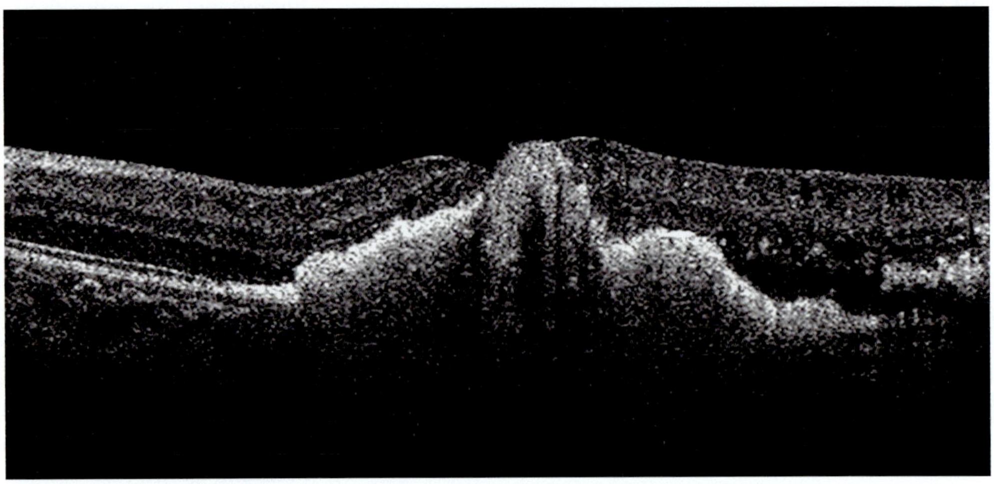

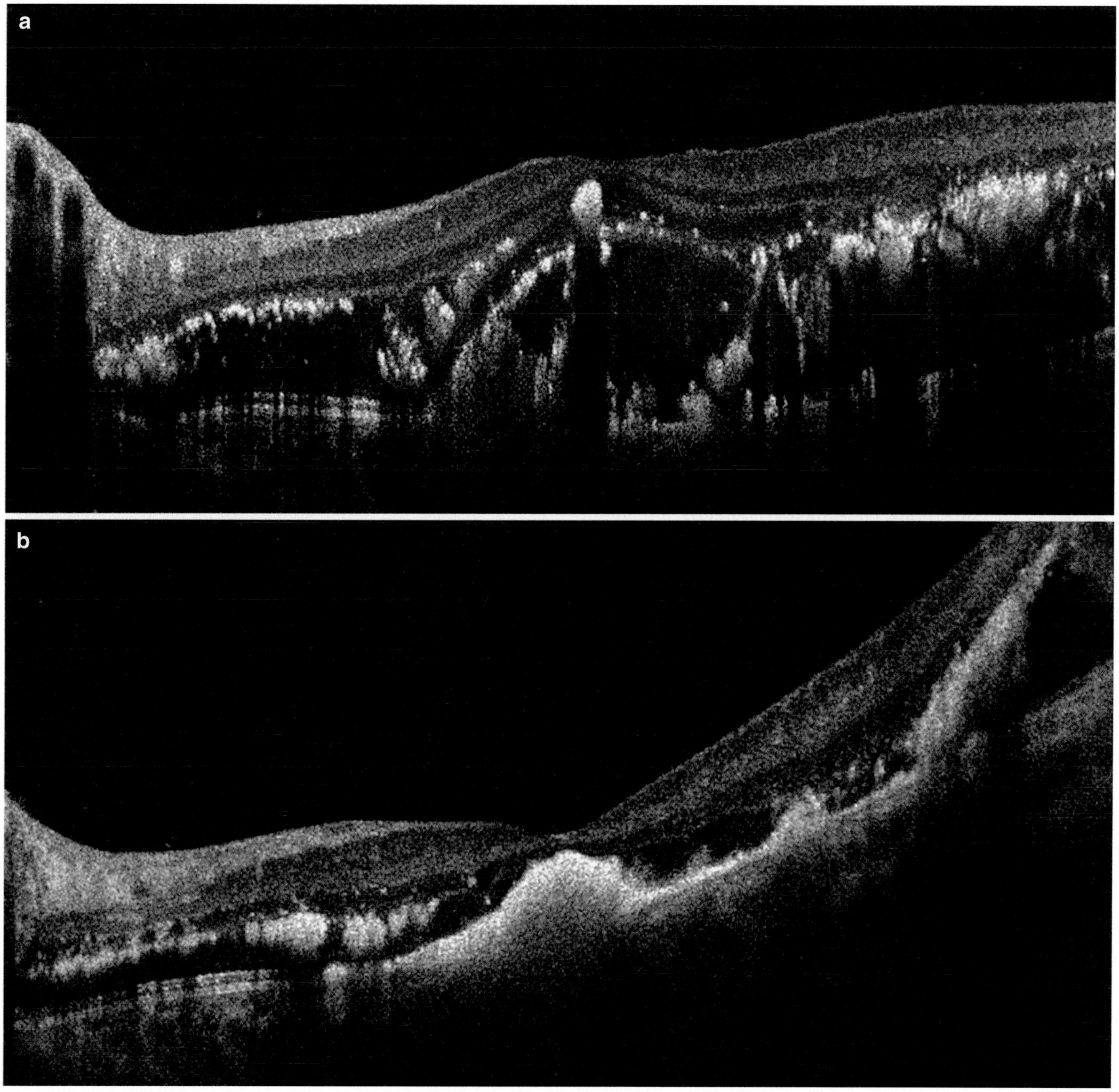

Fig. 8.7 Spectral domain optical coherence tomography images before (**a**, top) and after (**b**, bottom) laser photocoagulation and intravitreal bevacizumab. There are significant intraretinal exudates with anatomic improvement post-treatment

image the deep vascular plexus. OCTA findings in Coats' disease include anomalous vessels in the foveal avascular zone, rarefied capillary networks, and superficial and deep vascular plexuses (Muakkassa et al. 2016; Yonekawa et al. 2016; Stanga et al. 2016). However, OCTA alone has not been found to be a valid substitute for information garnered from FA (Hautz et al. 2017). Most importantly, OCTA does not yet show leakage, which FA does. From a practical standpoint, OCTA for Coats' disease is challenging for a number of reasons: (1) OCTA requires good fixation, and if the macula is involved, which is usually the case, steady fixation would be challenging for the patient, (2) pediatric patients are less likely to be as cooperative as adults during imaging sessions, and (3) current OCTA technologies are not wide angle, and require steering to image peripheral pathology. This, compounded by the patient age and poor fixation, limits the image quality and feasibility in most patients. The technology is ever evolving, however, and future devices may allow OCTA to play a larger role in Coats' disease management. At the time of writing, WFA and OCT in combination are the synergistic studies that provide the most important information for the diagnosis and management of Coats' disease.

Management

Non-surgical Interventions

The primary goals in Coats' disease treatment are to eliminate the telangiectatic vessels and aneurysms to resolve retinal exudation (Shields et al. 2001a). Laser photocoagulation is used as first-line treatment. Laser photocoagulation treatment is often combined with other therapeutics for severe disease, such as intravitreal anti-vascular endothelial growth factor (VEGF) injections, but is the most effective and definitive treatment (Munira et al. 2013; Grosso et al. 2015; Ghorbanian et al. 2012). Cryotherapy is also an ablative therapy and decreases the risk for further exudation and retinal detachment, but has a higher risk of potential complications, such as further exudation and hyaloidal contraction (Budning et al. 1998; Ghorbanian et al. 2012; Sigler et al. 2014). Laser treatment therefore is the first-line treatment as it can more directly and focally treat the lesions, and provide gentler peripheral ablation in the avascular retina.

Several lasering approaches can be employed when treating eyes with Coats' disease. Yellow or green lasers are recommended in order to penetrate through the exudation. Scatter laser is applied to the avascular retina and telangiectasia in a near confluent fashion. Aneurysms also need to be focally ablated, and usually require multiple applications of the laser on repeat or continuous mode. Care must be taken not to create iatrogenic breaks, which may occur with laser burns that are too intense. Often times, there is subretinal fluid present that prevents optimal laser uptake. Thankfully in Coats' disease, we are treating focal retinal vasculature and not the underlying retinal pigment epithelium, so we can "paint" the diseased vasculature and aneurysms with laser, usually on continuous mode or long burns. This alone can resolve the subretinal fluid and exudation. Laser treatment can also be supplemented with anti-VEGF and steroid treatment.

Although retinal peripheral nonperfusion is commonly found in Coats' disease, neovascularization of the retina or the optic nerve is interestingly uncommon. The ischemic retina is thought to upregulate VEGF secretion, quantified by reports of increased concentrations of VEGF in the vitreous of diseased eyes, resulting in increased vascular permeability of the telangiectatic vessels and exudation (Sun et al. 2007; He et al. 2010; Kase et al. 2013; Zhao et al. 2014). This fact supports a role for anti-VEGF therapeutics in the treatment of Coats'. Anti-VEGF injections are usually adjunctive therapies and are particularly useful in cases where subretinal fluid precludes definitive ablative therapy. The most commonly used anti-VEGF therapeutic is bevacizumab, followed by ranibizumab (Giannakopoulos et al. 2016; Gaillard et al. 2014). Both are off-label indications, and detailed informed consent is recommended. Many reports demonstrate that bevacizumab in combination with laser photocoagulation achieves near-complete or complete resolution of retinal exudation and detachments (Villegas et al. 2014; Kodama et al. 2014; Stergiou et al. 2009; Ray et al. 2013; Lin et al. 2010).

Corticosteroid intravitreal or periocular injections are also used as an adjunctive therapy in the management of Coats' disease. Steroids, such as triamcinolone, are thought to stabilize the blood-retinal microcirculation and thus improve vascular permeability (Tripathi and Ashton 1971). Similar to anti-VEGF agents, steroids are predominantly used to help decrease subretinal fluid prior to more definitive laser ablation of telangiectatic vessels (Jarin et al. 2005; Othman et al. 2010). However, steroids are not without complications, including cataract formation and the development of glaucoma; as many as 40% of Coats' eyes require cataract surgery following intravitreal triamcinolone (Othman et al. 2010).

Surgical Intervention

Surgical intervention is usually reserved for advanced cases of Coats' disease, as large exudative detachments often require surgical drainage. In these cases, internal drainage retinotomies during vitrectomy are generally avoided as this may result in proliferative vitreoretinopathy, and practically speaking, the subretinal exudation may not be able to be completely aspirated out for retinopexy of the retinotomy (Sigler et al. 2014; Imaizumi et al. 2016). Surgical methods for exudative retinal detachments from Coats' disease include trans-zonular infusion through a trocar placed in the anterior chamber and transscleral external drainage of subretinal exudation to facilitate indirect laser photocoagulation. If this is not sufficient, the external drainage may be facilitated with vitrectomy and perfluoro-n-octane (PFO), which can steamroll the fluid out through the sclerotomy, and allow the surgeon to apply endolaser (Fig. 8.8) (Imaizumi et al. 2016; Karacorlu et al. 2017; Muftuoglu and Gulkilik 2011;

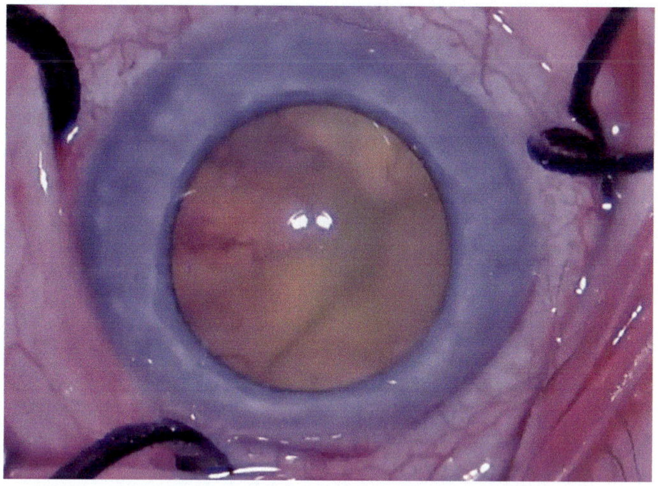

Fig. 8.8 Total retinal detachment from Coats' disease. This eye was treated with trans-zonular infusion, external drainage of subretinal exudates facilitated by vitrectomy and perfluoro-n-octane, and endolaser application (Image courtesy of Antonio Capone Jr, MD)

Adam and Kertes 2007; Mrejen et al. 2008; Yoshizumi et al. 1995; Suesskind et al. 2014). Silicone oil may sometimes be required for recurrent bullous exudation. Although visual prognosis remains guarded in eyes with advanced disease necessitating surgery, innovations in surgical intervention have provided globe-salvaging options and helped prevent progression to end-stage pathology, such as neovascular glaucoma and phthisis bulbi.

References

Adam RS, Kertes PJ. Observations on the management of Coats' disease: less is more. Br J Ophthalmol. 2007;91(3):303–6.

Anderson BH, Kasher PR, Mayer J, Szynkiewicz M, Jenkinson EM, Bhaskar SS, et al. Mutations in CTC1, encoding conserved telomere maintenance component 1, cause Coats plus. Nat Genet. 2012;44(3):338–42.

Blair MP, Ulrich JN, Elizabeth Hartnett M, Shapiro MJ. Peripheral retinal nonperfusion in fellow eyes in coats disease. Retina. 2013;33(8):1694–9.

Budning AS, Heon E, Gallie BL. Visual prognosis of Coats' disease. J AAPOS. 1998;2(6):356–9.

Char DH. Coats' syndrome: long term follow up. Br J Ophthalmol. 2000;84(1):37–9.

Coats G. Forms of retinal diseases with massive exudation. Roy Lond Ophthalmol Hosp Rep. 1908;17:440–525.

Daruich AL, Moulin AP, Tran HV, Matet A, Munier FL. Subfoveal nodule in Coats' disease: toward an updated classification predicting visual prognosis. Retina. 2017;37(8):1591–8.

Egerer I, Tasman W, Tomer TL. Coats disease. Arch Ophthalmol. 1974;92(2):109–12.

Gaillard M-C, Mataftsi A, Balmer A, Houghton S, Munier FL. Ranibizumab in the management of advanced Coats disease stages 3B and 4: long-term outcomes. Retina. 2014;34(11):2275–81.

Ganesh A, Kaliki S, Shields CL. Coats-like retinopathy in an infant with preclinical facioscapulohumeral dystrophy. J AAPOS. 2012;16(2):204–6.

Ghorbanian S, Jaulim A, Chatziralli IP. Diagnosis and treatment of Coats' disease: a review of the literature. Ophthalmologica. 2012;227(4):175–82.

Giannakopoulos M, Drimtzias E, Panteli V, Vasilakis P, Gartaganis SP. Intravitreal ranibizumab as an adjunctive treatment for Coats disease (6-year follow-up). Retin Cases Brief Rep. 2016;28

Gomez Morales A. Coats' disease. Natural history and results of treatment. Am J Ophthalmol. 1965;60(5):855–65.

Grosso A, Pellegrini M, Cereda MG, Panico C, Staurenghi G, Sigler EJ. Pearls and pitfalls in diagnosis and management of coats disease. Retina. 2015;35(4):614–23.

Hautz W, Gołębiewska J, Kocyła-Karczmarewicz B. Optical coherence tomography and optical coherence tomography angiography in monitoring Coats' disease. J Ophthalmol. 2017;2017:7849243.

He Y-G, Wang H, Zhao B, Lee J, Bahl D, McCluskey J. Elevated vascular endothelial growth factor level in Coats' disease and possible therapeutic role of bevacizumab. Graefes Arch Clin Exp Ophthalmol. 2010;248(10):1519–21.

Imaizumi A, Kusaka S, Takaesu S, Sawaguchi S, Shimomura Y. Subretinal fluid drainage and vitrectomy are helpful in diagnosing and treating eyes with advanced Coats' disease. Case Rep Ophthalmol. 2016;7(1):223–9.

Jarin RR, Teoh SCB, Lim TH. Resolution of severe macular oedema in adult Coat's syndrome with high-dose intravitreal triamcinolone acetonide. Eye. 2005;20(2):163–5.

Jeng-Miller KW, Gupta M, Rao P, Chan RP, Capone A, Mukai S, et al. Fellow eye findings in Coats' disease: longitudinal serial evaluation with widefield fluorescein angiography. Poster presented at The Retina Society, Boston, MA; 6 Oct 2017.

Jumper JM, Pomerleau D, McDonald HR, Johnson RN, Fu AD, Cunningham ET. Macular fibrosis in Coats disease. Retina. 2010;30(4 Suppl):S9–14.

Kang KB, Wessel MM, Tong J, D'Amico DJ, Chan RVP. Ultra-widefield imaging for the management of pediatric retinal diseases. J Pediatr Ophthalmol Strabismus. 2013;50(5):282–8.

Karacorlu M, Hocaoglu M, Sayman Muslubas I, Arf S. Long-term anatomical and functional outcomes following vitrectomy for advanced coats disease. Retina. 2017;37(9):1757–64.

Kase S, Rao NA, Yoshikawa H, Fukuhara J, Noda K, Kanda A, et al. Expression of vascular endothelial growth factor in eyes with Coats' disease. Invest Ophthalmol Vis Sci. 2013;54(1):57–62.

Khurana RN, Samuel MA, Murphree AL, Loo RH, Tawansy KA. Subfoveal nodule in Coats' disease. Clin Exp Ophthalmol. 2005;33(3):301–2.

Kodama A, Sugioka K, Kusaka S, Matsumoto C, Shimomura Y. Combined treatment for Coats' disease: retinal laser photocoagulation combined with intravitreal bevacizumab injection was effective in two cases. BMC Ophthalmol. 2014;14:36.

Leber T. Ueber Vorkommen durch eine Form von multipler Miliaraneurysmen charakterisierte Retinaldegeneration. F Arch Ophthalmol. 1912;81:1–14.

Lin C-J, Hwang J-F, Chen Y-T, Chen S-N. The effect of intravitreal bevacizumab in the treatment of Coats disease in children. Retina. 2010;30(4):617–22.

Mrejen S, Metge F, Denion E, Dureau P, Edelson C, Caputo G. Management of retinal detachment in Coats disease. Study of 15 cases. Retina. 2008;28(3 Suppl):S26–32.

Muakkassa NW, de Carlo TE, Choudhry N, Duker JS, Baumal CR. Optical coherence tomography angiography findings in Coats' disease. Ophthalmic Surg Lasers Imaging Retina. 2016;47(7):632–5.

Mufuoglu G, Gulkilik G. Pars plana vitrectomy in advanced Coats' disease. Case Rep Ophthalmol. 2011;2(1):15–22.

Munira Y, Zunaina E, Azhany Y. Resolution of exudative retinal detachment and regression of retinal macrocyst post-laser in Coats disease. Int Med Case Rep J. 2013;6:37–9.

Ong SS, Buckley EG, McCuen BW, Jaffe GJ, Postel EA, Mahmoud TH, et al. Comparison of visual outcomes in Coats' disease: a 20-year experience. Ophthalmology. 2017;28. pii: S0161-6420(16)32449-6.

Othman IS, Moussa M, Bouhaimed M. Management of lipid exudates in Coats disease by adjuvant intravitreal triamcinolone: effects and complications. Br J Ophthalmol. 2010;94(5):606–10.

Ray R, Barañano DE, Hubbard GB. Treatment of Coats' disease with intravitreal bevacizumab. Br J Ophthalmol. 2013;97(3):272–7.

Reese AB. Telangiectasis of the retina and Coats' disease. Am J Ophthalmol. 1956;42(1):1–8.

Ridley ME, Shields JA, Brown GC, Tasman W. Coats' disease. Evaluation of management. Ophthalmology. 1982;89(12):1381–7.

Shane TS, Berrocal AM, Hess DJ. Bilateral fluorescein angiographic findings in unilateral Coats' disease. Ophthalmic Surg Lasers Imaging. 2011;42. Online:e15–7.

Shields JA, Shields CL. Review: coats disease: the 2001 LuEsther T. Mertz lecture. Retina. 2002;22(1):80–91.

Shields JA, Shields CL, Honavar SG, Demirci H. Clinical variations and complications of Coats disease in 150 cases: the 2000 Sanford Gifford Memorial Lecture. Am J Ophthalmol. 2001a;131(5):561–71.

Shields JA, Shields CL, Honavar SG, Demirci H, Cater J. Classification and management of Coats disease: the 2000 Proctor Lecture. Am J Ophthalmol. 2001b;131(5):572–83.

Sigler EJ, Randolph JC, Calzada JI, Wilson MW, Haik BG. Current management of Coats disease. Surv Ophthalmol. 2014;59(1):30–46.

Stanga PE, Papayannis A, Tsamis E, Chwiejczak K, Stringa F, Jalil A, et al. Swept-source optical coherence tomography angiography of paediatric macular diseases. Dev Ophthalmol. 2016;56:166–73.

Statland JM, Sacconi S, Farmakidis C, Donlin-Smith CM, Chung M, Tawil R. Coats syndrome in facioscapulohumeral dystrophy type 1: frequency and D4Z4 contraction size. Neurology. 2013;80(13):1247–50.

Stergiou PK, Symeonidis C, Dimitrakos SA. Coats' disease: treatment with intravitreal bevacizumab and laser photocoagulation. Acta Ophthalmol. 2009;87(6):687–8.

Suesskind D, Altpeter E, Schrader M, Bartz-Schmidt KU, Aisenbrey S. Pars plana vitrectomy for treatment of advanced Coats' disease–presentation of a modified surgical technique and long-term follow-up. Graefes Arch Clin Exp Ophthalmol. 2014;252(6):873–9.

Sun Y, Jain A, Moshfeghi DM. Elevated vascular endothelial growth factor levels in Coats disease: rapid response to pegaptanib sodium. Graefes Arch Clin Exp Ophthalmol. 2007;245(9):1387–8.

Tarkkanen A, Laatikainen L. Coat's disease: clinical, angiographic, histopathological findings and clinical management. Br J Ophthalmol. 1983;67(11):766–76.

Tolmie JL, Browne BH, McGettrick PM, Stephenson JB. A familial syndrome with Coats' reaction retinal angiomas, hair and nail defects and intracranial calcification. Eye. 1988;2(Pt 3):297–303.

Tripathi R, Ashton N. Electron microscopical study of Coat's disease. Br J Ophthalmol. 1971;55(5):289–301.

Vance SK, Wald KJ, Sherman J, Freund KB. Subclinical facioscapulohumeral muscular dystrophy masquerading as bilateral Coats disease in a woman. Arch Ophthalmol. 2011;129(6):807–9.

Villegas VM, Gold AS, Berrocal AM, Murray TG. Advanced Coats' disease treated with intravitreal bevacizumab combined with laser vascular ablation. Clin Ophthalmol. 2014;8:973–6.

Yannuzzi NA, Tzu JH, Ko AC, Hess DJ, Cristian I, Berrocal AM. Ocular findings and treatment of a young boy with Coats' plus. Ophthalmic Surg Lasers Imaging Retina. 2014;45(5):462–5.

Yonekawa Y, Todorich B, Trese MT. Optical coherence tomography angiography findings in Coats' disease. Ophthalmology. 2016;123(9):1964.

Yoshizumi MO, Kreiger AE, Lewis H, Foxman B, Hakakha BA. Vitrectomy techniques in late-stage Coats'-like exudative retinal detachment. Doc Ophthalmol. 1995;90(4):387–94.

Zhao Q, Peng X-Y, Chen F-H, Zhang Y-P, Wang L, You Q-S, et al. Vascular endothelial growth factor in Coats' disease. Acta Ophthalmol. 2014;92(3):e225–8.

Paediatric Retinal Inflammatory Disorders

9

Jessy Choi, Alexander Bossuyt, Nicole Shu-Wen Chan, and Grace Wu

Abbreviations

APMPPE	Acute posterior multifocal placoid pigment epitheliopathy
ARN	Acute retinal necrosis
AC	Ampiginous choroiditis
ACE	Angiotensin-converting enzyme
anti-VEGF	Anti-vascular endothelial growth factor
BCG	Bacillus Calmette-Guérin
BD	Behçet disease
B-scan	Brightness scan
CARD15	Caspase recruitment domain-containing protein 15
CSD	Cat scratch disease
CDC	Centre for Disease Control
CNS	Central nervous system
CD4	Cluster of differentiation 4
CMV	Cytomegalovirus
DNA	Deoxyribonucleic acid
DMARD	Disease-modifying antirheumatic drug
EOCS	Early-onset childhood sarcoidosis
EBE	Endogenous bacterial endophthalmitis
ELISA	Enzyme-linked immunosorbent assay
EBV	Epstein Barr Virus
FFA	Fluorescein fundus angiography
HHV	Human herpes virus
HIV	Human Immunodeficiency virus
HLA-B51	Human leucocyte antigen B51
HLA	Human leukocyte antigens
HSV-1	Human simplex virus type 1
HSV-2	Human simplex virus type 2
HTLV-1	Human T-cell lymphoma virus type 1
IRVAN	Idiopathic retinal vasculitis, aneurysms, and neuroretinitis
NOD2	nucleotide binding oligomerization domain 2
PRP	Pan retinal photocoagulation
PORN	Progressive outer retinal necrosis
RPE	Retinal pigment epithelium
SO	Sympathetic ophthalmia
T. Gondii	*Toxoplasma gondii*
UK	United Kingdom
VZV	Varicella-zoster virus
VDRL	Venereal disease research laboratory
VKH	Vogt–Koyanagi–Harada

J. Choi (✉)
Department of Ophthalmology, Sheffield Children's Hospital NHS Foundation Trust, Sheffield, UK
e-mail: jessy.choi@nhs.net

A. Bossuyt
University of Nottingham, Nottingham, UK

N. S.-W. Chan · G. Wu
Department of Ophthalmology, National University Hospital, Singapore, Singapore
e-mail: grace.wu.y.m@singhealth.com.sg

Introduction

Inflammatory disease affecting the retina in children is a rare and potentially blinding condition, with a diverse etiology. It encompasses a spectrum of disorders of the posterior segment, and may also be labelled as posterior uveitis, chorioretinitis, retinal vasculitis, retinitis, or retinal necrosis. Inflammatory retinal disease may occur in isolation or in association with a systemic condition. It is vital to differentiate an infectious etiology, especially in children that are immunocompromised, as the diagnosis always has profound implications systemically. Immunocompetent neonates with features indicative of congenital cytomegalovirus or toxoplasmosis are often asymptomatic and referred for target screening by a neonatologist.

The presenting symptoms of retinitis can vary greatly in children. It can range from asymptomatic to a painful red eye with profound sight loss. Symptoms of pain tend to present in infective causes. Other presenting symptoms may be subtle such as a mild red eye, complaints of photophobia, floaters, or blurry vision in older verbal children, especially when both eyes are involved.

Inflammation of the retina can affect the veins and/or the arterioles. It is described as a fluffy perivascular white cuff of

R. V. P. Chan (ed.), *Pediatric Retinal Diseases*, Retina Atlas, https://doi.org/10.1007/978-981-19-1364-8_9

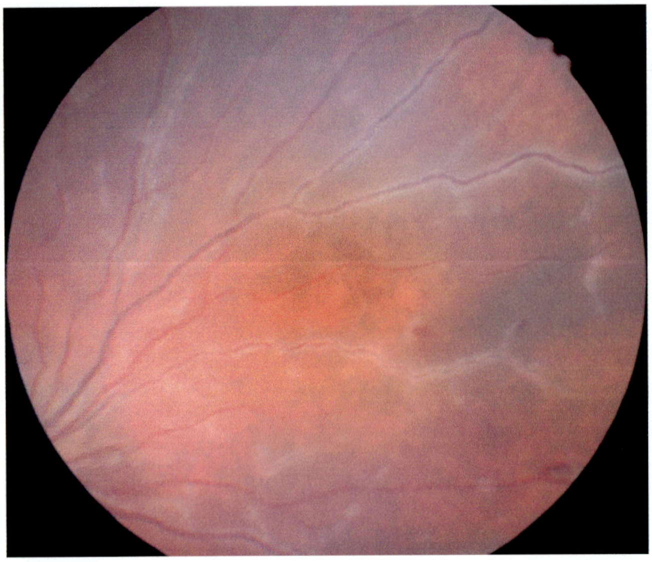

Fig. 9.1 Colour fundus image of the right eye demonstrating extensive inflammation of the retinal vessels predominantly affecting the vein demonstrating the appearance of periphlebitis

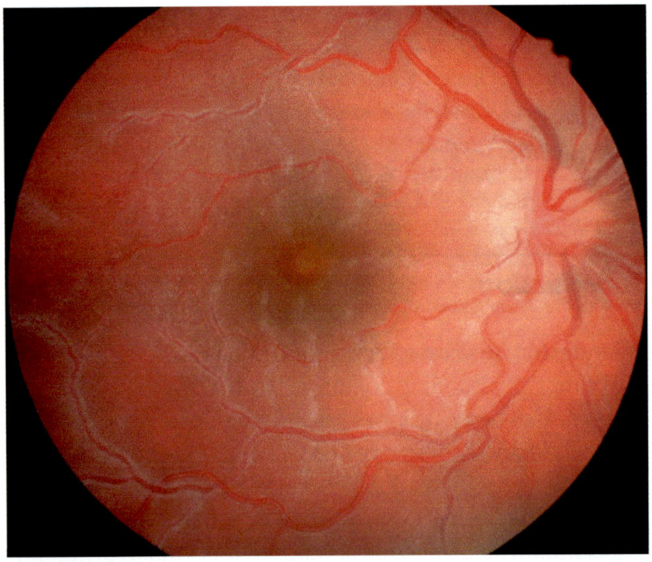

Fig. 9.2 Colour fundus image of the right eye demonstrating extensive macular oedema secondary to widespread retinal vasculitis affecting mainly the venous system. This image is from a 12-year-old girl with idiopathic bilateral retinal vasculitis with a vision reduced to Logmar 1.2. She underwent extensive systemic workup and responded excellently to systemic immunomodulation and steroids. Her vision improved to Logmar 0.05; 6 months after initial presentation

exudation during the active stage (Fig. 9.1) with associated intraretinal haemorrhage, oedema (Fig. 9.2), and retinal artery or vein occlusion leading to retinal ischaemia (Fig. 9.3) with cotton wool spots (Fig. 9.4) and the formation of micro or macro aneurysms.

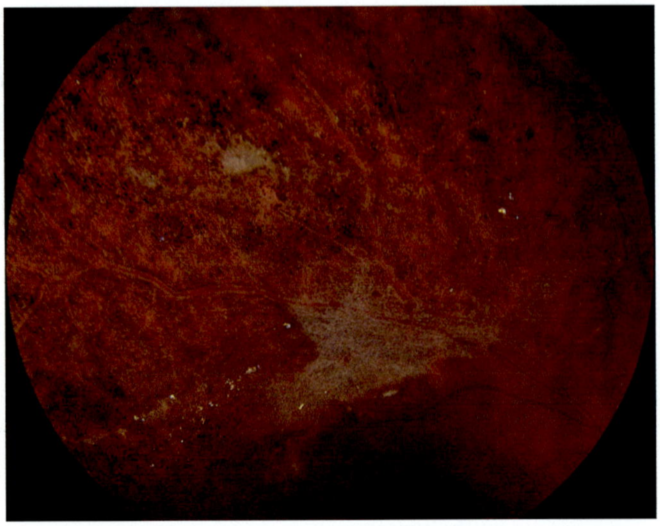

Fig. 9.3 Colour fundus image of a young boy with treated CMV retinitis demonstrating areas of retinal atrophy, vascular occlusion, and tractional retinal membrane. The subtle, thin, non-fluffy outline of perivascular sheathing can be seen during mild or inactive periods

Assessment of the extent of retinal vasculitis requires investigations such as fluorescein angiography or indocyanine green angiography to demarcate the avascular ischaemic areas, and to detect active disease that may not be visible clinically, particularly at the extreme periphery (Fig. 9.5). Ocular coherence tomography (OCT) is useful to detect subclinical macular oedema (Fig. 9.6) and tractional retinopathy.

These investigations can pose their own challenges in young children. Cooperation from young patients can be tricky when trying to capture angiograms in a timely manner. In addition, paediatric specialists with experience in paediatric resuscitation need to be on standby when performing any intravenous injection of dye in case of fatal anaphylactic shock.

If it is not possible to do these investigations with cooperation from the child alternative measures may be considered, such as performing the procedures under sedation or general anaesthesia in centres with an ultra-wide-field supine fundus imaging system. Otherwise, oral fluorescein can be considered in select older children, and angiography can be obtained with an adult non-contact confocal scanning laser ophthalmoscopy imaging system.

The visual prognosis of inflammatory conditions of the retina in children can vary greatly due to the wide variety of causes. Proactive rapid management is essential, especially to prevent involvement of the contralateral eye when patients present with unilateral infective retinitis. Children with retinitis are almost always best managed with a multi-disciplinary approach.

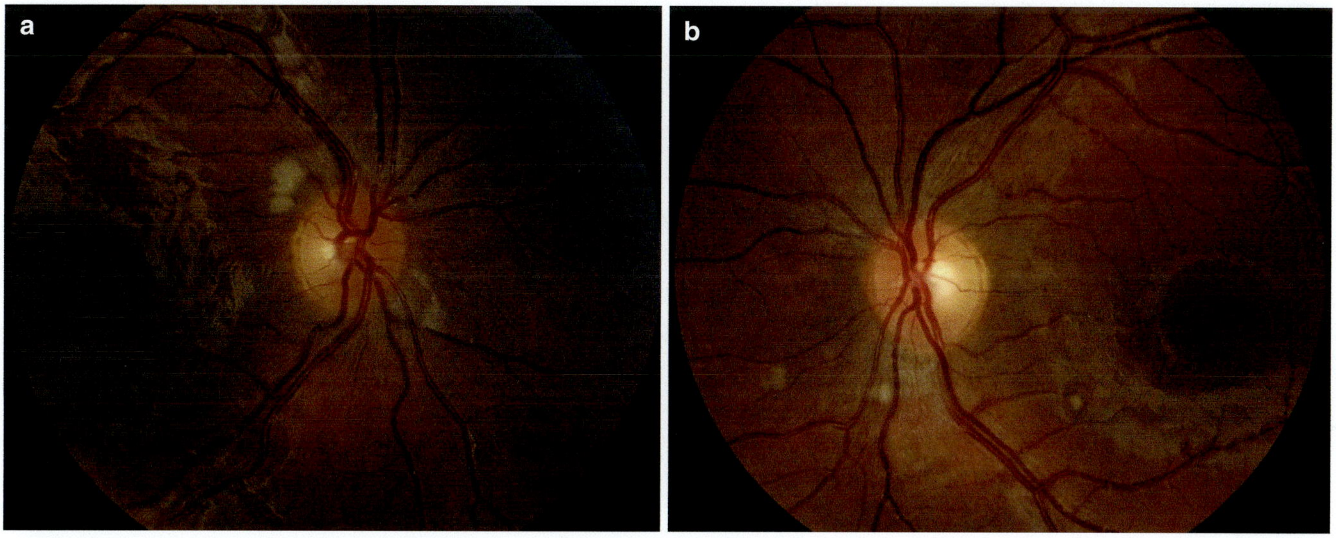

Fig. 9.4 (**a**) and (**b**) Colour fundus image of the right and left retina showing cotton wool spots in a 12-year-old with systemic vasculitis

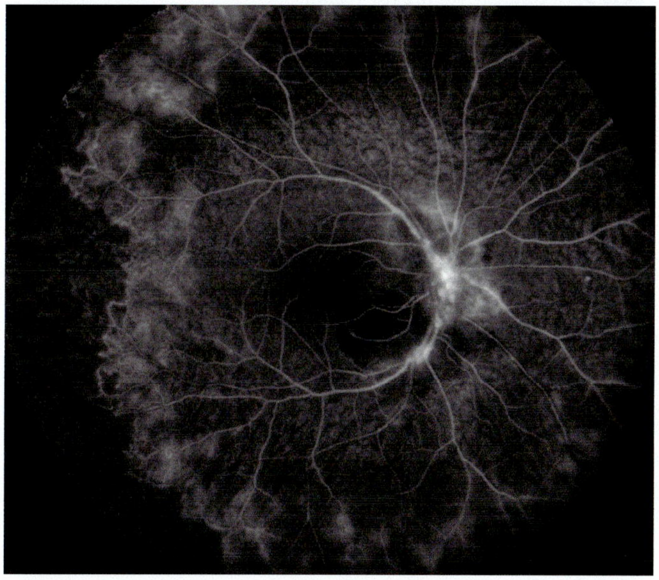

Fig. 9.5 Fluorescein fundus angiography (FFA) of the right eye taken from a 13-year-old with idiopathic retinal vasculitis, aneurysms, and neuroretinitis (IRVAN) showing peripheral vascular non-perfusion demonstrated in this late phase oral FFA (weight adjusted)

Clinical Entities

Infectious

Bacteria

It is crucial to make a diagnosis of bacterial retinitis early, so specific antibiotics can be started promptly to save sight and life. Treating the infective retinitis with anti-inflammatory therapy alone can be damaging.

Tuberculosis

Mycobacterium tuberculosis is responsible for most human tuberculosis (TB). It is a gram-positive acid-fast bacillus. The World Health Organization estimates one-third of the world population (approximately 2 billion people) (World Health Organization 2013) are infected with TB, with 9 million new cases diagnosed each year, 95% of new cases are found in developing countries. TB kills more than 1 million individuals each year. Approximately 5% of infected individuals develop clinical TB within 2 years from initial exposure (Zumla et al. 2013) with only 10% being symptomatic, in which 80% have pulmonary features (Shakarchi 2015). The increased incidence of TB worldwide in both developing and developed countries is linked to multidrug-resistance (Gandhi et al. 2010), human immunodeficiency virus (HIV), global migration, immunosuppressive therapies, socioeconomic status, and poverty (Hawker et al. 1999).

In a North India study, TB was identified in 15% of all paediatric uveitis patients; 44% were reported as posterior uveitis (Gautam et al. 2018).

TB uveitis is typically granulomatous with mutton fat keratic precipitates and par planitis ± snowballs. Choroidal granuloma with exudative retinal detachment is commonly reported in systemic TB. Serpiginous like choroiditis is more common among young and middle-aged patients from TB endemic areas e.g. Asia Pacific (Ganesh et al. 2016). Retinal haemorrhagic periphlebitis with exudative and occlusive retinal vasculitis is highly suggestive of TB (Desai et al. 2020). Other ocular findings include pan-ophthalmitis, endophthalmitis, papillitis, neuroretinitis, and optic nerve tubercle.

The diagnosis of TB is made by taking an accurate travel and contact history, systemic findings, suggestive ocular

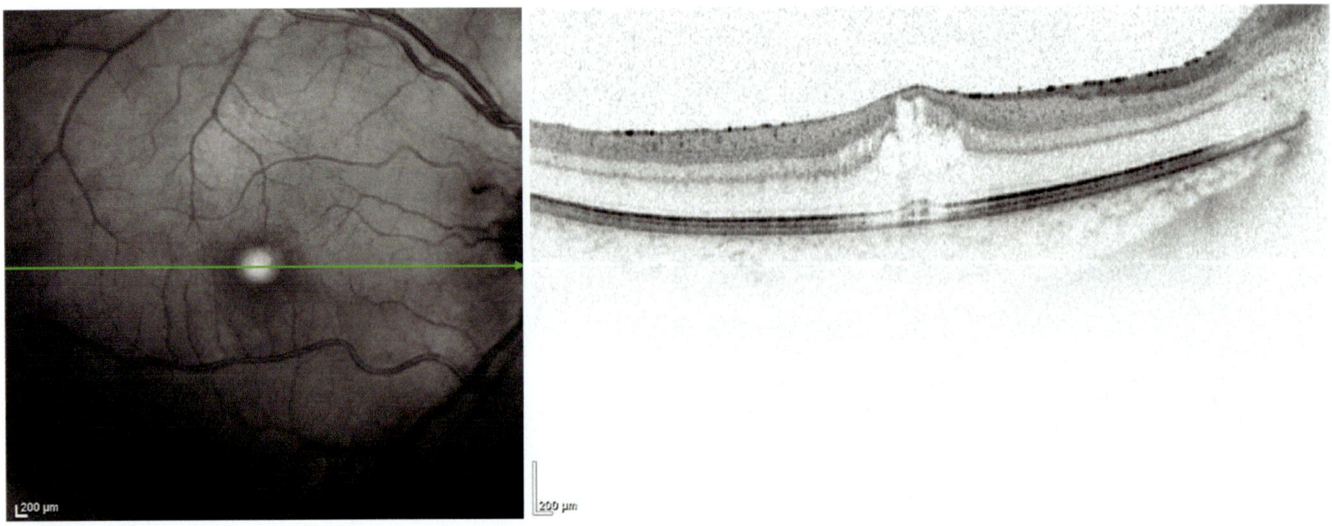

Fig. 9.6 OCT of a 5-year-old with cystoid macular oedema secondary to vitritis and toxocariasis

findings, and the result of investigations such as chest X-ray, tuberculin skin test, interferon-gamma release assays (e.g. QuantiFERON), and a positive response to anti-tuberculosis treatment. The tuberculin skin test is not specific for differentiating false-positive results from previous exposure to Bacillus Calmette-Guérin (BCG) vaccination; however, the effect declines after 7 years, therefore a strong positive tuberculin test is unlikely to be caused by the BCG vaccine. Polymerase chain reaction (PCR) is useful in detecting TB, specifically in an intraocular sample, although it can lack sensitivity (Shakarchi 2015; Ang et al. 2018; Gupta et al. 2007).

The management of children with TB must involve paediatric infectious disease specialists to optimize outcomes in the use of systemic anti-TB therapy, e.g. isoniazid, rifampicin, ethambutol, pyrazinamide, or pyroxidine (Figueira et al. 2017).

Syphilis

Treponema Pallidum is a small helical flagellated spirochete bacterium, typically sexually transmitted by contact with active mucocutaneous lesions. Spirochetes penetrate intact mucosal surfaces directly; then trigger a T-lymphocyte mediated response. The incidence of syphilis reduced during the latter part of the twentieth century due to effective antibacterial treatment but is on the rise in the past 15 years, particularly affecting metropolitan areas, potentially due to the fall in the use of barrier protection (condoms), especially in male homosexual populations. This can be seen in the change of gender polarity towards male with the ratio between male and female shown to be 5:1 in the United Kingdom (UK) (Braxton et al. 2018; Simms et al. 2005).

Syphilis in children can be congenital via vertical transmission trans-placentally to the foetus. It is rare, but on the rise, with the Centre for Disease Control (CDC) reporting in 2017 that the rate of congenital syphilis has increased each year since 2012, in 2017, there was a rate of 23.3 cases per 100,000 births in the USA (Braxton et al. 2018). Sexually active children can acquire syphilis like in adults with abuse being of particular concern (Arnold and Ford-Jones 2000).

Table 9.1 Clinical staging for syphilis

Stage 1	Occurs 3 weeks after exposure and is characterized by painless ulcerative chancre at the contact points and regional lymphadenopathy
Stage 2	Occurs 2–12 weeks after exposure with arthralgia, pyrexia, malaise, maculopapular rash, painless generalized lymphadenopathy and highly infectious condylomata mucosae lesions.
Stage 3	Occurs months to years after stage 2, focal gummatous inflammation involving the eye, aorta, and neurosyphilis.

Paediatric syphilis shares a similar clinical picture with adult syphilis with three stages of systemic manifestations if left untreated (See Table 9.1).

Ocular involvement occurs in the latent phase of stages 2 and 3 and is a great mimicker with a wide variety of clinical features. Syphilis commonly involves the posterior segment with an incidence of 3/100,000. Panuveitis is the commonest sign in 40% of cases (Mathew et al. 2014). Eyelid chancre is rare and found in primary syphilis. Condylomata lata are skin lesions on the eyelid with widespread involvement of the face, which often occur in secondary syphilis (Mets and Chhabra 2008).

Anterior segment involvement varies from stromal keratitis, iridocyclitis, granulomatous or non-granulomatous iris nodules. Dilated iris capillaries (iris roseola) are highly suggestive of syphilitic infections. Interstitial keratitis and ghost vessels are usually found in congenital cases (Mets and Chhabra 2008).

Posterior segment involvement varies from multifocal chorioretinitis, retinal necrosis (especially in those with coexisting HIV), punctate inner neuroretinitis, subretinal neovascular membrane, retinal vasculitis, macular oedema, pseudo retinitis pigmentosa (salt and pepper appearance), vitritis, disc oedema, serous effusion, retinal detachment, and central retinal artery occlusion. Acute syphilitic posterior placoid chorioretinitis described by Gass is reported to be highly suggestive of syphilis (Gass et al. 1990). It consists of large white oval placoid lesions covering the whole macular. Coinfection with HIV can give an atypical presentation, such as isolated vitritis (Kuo et al. 1998).

Neurosyphilis involvement varies from Argyll-Robertson pupil, optic neuropathy, bitemporal hemianopia, cortical blindness, and gaze palsies (Mets and Chhabra 2008).

Congenital syphilis can manifest clinically at various times throughout life, typically salt and pepper chorioretinitis, glaucoma, and uveitis are commonly found below the age of 1, while interstitial keratitis tends to occur after the age 1 (Arnold and Ford-Jones 2000).

The diagnosis of *Treponema Pallidum* can be made with direct visualization by using dark field techniques in tissue sampling, and serological testing. Non-treponemal tests are used to detect cardiolipin-lecithin-cholesterol antigen antibodies in a venereal disease research laboratory (VDRL). Enzyme-linked immunosorbent assay (ELISA) is used to specifically detect treponemal antigens. PCR can be used for analysing intraocular tissue biopsies.

Treatment of syphilis in children involves close collaboration with paediatric infectious disease specialists, the treatment typically includes high-dose systemic penicillin (Arnold and Ford-Jones 2000). Uveitis is often being treated as neurosyphilis, with a more prolonged course of systemic antibacterial agents alongside topical steroids.

Lyme (Borreliosis)

Lyme disease is the most common human tick-borne disease in the Northern hemisphere and is caused by *Borrelia*. The spirochete bacterium was first described by Willy Burgdorfer in 1981. There are now 40 distinct species with marked diversity causing Lyme disease, these species are grouped under *Borrelia burgdorferi*. It is named after Old Lyme in Connecticut USA in 1975 (Nelson and Williams 2007). The disease is most prevalent in forest and heathland, e.g. New England in North America and parts of Europe. Lyme is transmitted to human by the bite of infected hard-bodied ticks, *Ixodes scapularis* in New England, *Ixodes pacificus* in mid-west USA, and *Ixodes ricinus* in Europe.

There is a large variance of incidence for Lyme disease, with rates as low as 0.001/100,000 in Italy to as high as 464/100,000 in Sweden, although most studies recommend establishing more concrete and well-conducted surveillance research to monitor the disease (Sykes and Makiello 2017). There is a large variance within the USA as well, although a general incidence of around 12/100,000 has been reported (Rochlin et al. 2019).

The disease commonly affects the skin, nervous system, joints, and heart. Ocular involvement is reported to be 4% in paediatric cases, and commonly presents with uveitis (Mora and Carta 2009).

The clinical course of the disease has three stages. The initial stage is erythema chronicum migrans, manifested within the first month at the bite site, found in 60–80% of infected cases, whereas history of tick bites is found in only 50%. If untreated, it progresses to stage 2, where approximately 60% develop arthropathy; and roughly 15% have central nervous system (CNS) involvement, also known as neuroborreliosis with symptoms of meningism, peripheral neuropathy and cranial nerve palsy causing double vision. Cardiovascular involvement such as myocarditis, pericarditis, and atrioventricular heart block have been reported. Late persistent third stage disease affects a minority of patients, it manifests as progressive arthritis and parenchymal inflammation in the brain and spinal cord with symptoms of ataxia, encephalopathy, and cognitive alteration such as psychosis; spinal cord compression can also lead to permanent paralysis in the advanced cases (Halperin 2015).

Most of the ocular diseases described are predominately linked to the American pathogen *Borrelia burgdorferi sensu stricto* and *Borrelia mayonii*; while in Eurasia *Borrelia garinii* and *Borrelia afzelii* are more predominant, with a lower incidence of uveitis despite high seropositivity in the at risk population (Mysterud et al. 2019).

Ocular inflammation can affect any part of the eye, mimicking other inflammatory conditions and can occur months to years after the appearance of erythema migrans. Retinal vasculitis is reported to be fairly common and intermediate uveitis is the most common ocular manifestation (Mikkilä et al. 2000). Other features include papillitis, neuroretinitis, papilloedema, and ischaemic optic neuropathy (Stanek et al. 2012). Other less common ocular signs are self-limiting conjunctivitis found in stage 1. Interstitial keratitis has been reported with peripheral corneal vascularisation (Mikkilä et al. 2000; Huppertz et al. 1999; Weinberg 2008).

The diagnosis of Lyme borreliosis is mainly based on clinical features, such as chronic anterior uveitis, intermediate uveitis, or retinal vasculitis in association with erythema migrans, arthropathy, or neurological defects, then confirmed with serological testing. ELISA has a 90–100% sensitivity when continent-specific species are targeted. However, due to cross-reaction with other spirochetes (e.g. *Treponema pallidum*) it may give a false-positive result; therefore, it should be done in conjunction with syphilis serology to help clarity. False positives may also occur in patients with *Epstein Barr Virus* (EBV) or *Cytomegalovirus* (CMV), as well as in those with positive rheumatoid factor or antinuclear factor. Hence, it needs to be interpreted alongside the clinical history and findings. Western blot is a more confirmatory serological tool, however only 1/3 are positive for IgM or IgG for *Borrelia burgdorferi* in the acute phase. PCR is highly specific but can only detect *Borrelia* deoxyribonucleic acid (DNA) when present, therefore <50% is found when the erythema migrans rash is present, as it could be weeks or months after the tick bite and spirochetes may no longer be found in the blood (Steere et al. 2008).

For early infection in children, oral penicillin may be given. Intravenous penicillin or ceftriaxone are recommended to treat those with intraocular involvement or those with a severe and advanced condition (Stanek et al. 2012). A multi-disciplinary team approach is essential when managing children with suspected Lyme disease.

Endogenous Bacterial Endophthalmitis

Endogenous bacterial endophthalmitis (EBE) is when bacteria spread to the eye via haematogenous spread, it is less common than exogenous bacterial endophthalmitis forming just 2–6% of all cases of endophthalmitis (Jackson et al. 2003). *Staphylococcus* and *Streptococcal* species are common causative organisms in the Western countries while *Klebsiella pneumonia* is the most common cause in the Eastern countries (Wong et al. 2000; Greenwald et al. 1986). EBE is rare with an incidence of 6–8% in the general public and 0.1–0.4% in children (Sadiq et al. 2015; Maitray et al. 2019).

EBE is a result of the dissemination of septic emboli crossing the blood ocular barrier to cause microbial proliferation and inflammation in ocular tissues, commonly in the choroid, retina, and vitreous. Most of the paediatric EBE data comes from reported cases. Compared with adult endogenous endophthalmitis, children have more pronounced systemic signs such as sepsis, fever, and bacteraemia (Garg et al. 1991). Neonatal EBE is worth a special mention. The risk factors for neonatal EBE are low birth weight, existing ROP disease, babies with bacteraemia, and babies in shock (Moshfeghi et al. 2011; Basu et al. 2013; Noyola et al. 2002).

The hallmark feature of EBE is vitreous involvement. The typical features include eyelid oedema, conjunctival injection, circumcorneal congestion, pain, photophobia, and the presence of floaters. Anterior chamber inflammation with hypopyon, absent red reflex, vitreous cells, and haze may also be present (Sadiq et al. 2015).

Anterior chamber involvement is common in EBE (Okada et al. 1994). There may be a poor view of the fundus due to the presence of exudates and vitreous haze. Other findings include corneal oedema, presence of iris nodules, and pupillary distortion secondary to synechiae formation (Dua et al. 2006; Khan et al. 2002).

The most reliable way of diagnosing systemic infection is by taking blood cultures on three consecutive days. Optical imaging such as a brightness scan (B-scan) can detect vitreous and choroidal abscesses, and retinal detachment. OCT can reveal intraretinal lesions and subretinal collections. PCR can be useful in confirming pathogens in vitreous samples (Sadiq et al. 2015).

Treatment for EBE is with high-dose intravenous and intravitreal antibiotics. Vitrectomies may be necessary in serious cases. Visual prognosis tends to be poor in neonates and variable in children (Sadiq et al. 2015; Basu et al. 2013).

Cat Scratch Disease

Cat scratch disease (CSD) was first described by Parinaud in 1889 as a chronic fever with preauricular lymphadenopathy and granulomatous conjunctivitis (Parinaud 1889). These symptoms were later termed as Parinaud oculoglandular syndrome, and a history of cat exposure was also noted.

CSD is caused by *Bartonella Henselae*, a small facultative intracellular gram-negative bacterium. The transmission is most commonly from cat scratch or bite but can spread via contact between cat saliva and open wounds. The disease consists of a gradual progressive regional lymphadenopathy with malaise and fever. The incidence of CSD has been shown to be highest in children aged 5–9 years of age (9.4 cases/100,000) (Nelson et al. 2016). Around 10% of CSD patients develop atypical CSD where there are either musculoskeletal, neurological, dermatological, hepatosplenic, or ophthalmic manifestations (Rolain et al. 2004; Gandhi et al. 2015). The incidence of ocular manifestations in CSD has been reported to be around 4.4% (Habot-Wilner et al. 2018).

Bartonella invades and colonizes mature erythrocytes and endothelial cells, leading to an inflammatory response. Spread to the eye is thought to be haematogenous (Harms and Dehio 2012). A red/brown non-tender papule usually appears 3–10 days after initial contact with regional lymphadenopathy occurring 1–3 weeks later (Batts and Demers 2004).

Decreased vision is the most common presenting ocular symptom, reported in 88%. A similar proportion of patients also had swollen discs at presentation. Roughly 2/3 of ocular CSD presents with neuroretinitis, CSD being the most common cause of neuroretinitis (Habot-Wilner et al. 2018; Abdelhakim and Rasool 2018).

Diagnosis is based on history and clinical features. Serology is the mainstay for diagnosis of CSD, a combination of IgG and IgM ELISA (Habot-Wilner et al. 2018). PCR can be used for tissue or pus samples, but research on the sensitivity of this varies largely due to different laboratory conditions, with ranges between 18 and 80% being reported (Allizond et al. 2019).

CSD can be self-limiting, treatment for ocular manifestations is stratified by vision. Azithromycin has been shown to be the most appropriate antibiotic for children with CSD, although trimethoprim or sulfamethoxazole are suggested if azithromycin is contraindicated (Shorbatli et al. 2018).

Rickettsioses

Rickettsioses is a worldwide zoonoses caused by obligate intracellular gram-negative bacteria, usually transmitted via bites from ticks, mites, lice, or fleas. The *Rickettsiaceae* family of bacteria causes rickettsioses, with different pathogenic species being present in different regions of the world. *Rickettsia ricketsii* is found in the Americas, *Rickettsia conorii* is found in Europe and Africa, *Rickettsia sibirica* is found in Asia, and *Rickettsia australis* is found in Australia. The disease usually occurs in late spring or summer. Rickettsioses caused by *Rickettsia rickettsii* is also caused Rocky Mountain spotted fever and most commonly affects children between the age 5 and 9 years. The incidence in the US is estimated to be 2.2 per million (Marshall et al. 2003; Valbuena 2013).

From the skin, *Rickettsia* spreads via the bloodstream to infect the endothelium and vascular smooth muscle cells and can rapidly spread from cell to cell. Spread to the eye is haematogenous and can cause inflammation within (Valbuena 2013).

Rickettsial disease tends to present with the triad of rash, fever, and headache and general malaise. A black skin lesion may develop at the site of the bite for some rickettsioses. Patients usually give a history of outdoor activities or tick attachment (Tomassone et al. 2018). The rash is typically maculopapular, affecting the soles and palms but sparing the face. Most patients recover without any sequalae, but it may result in life-threatening complications such as meningoencephalitis (Carvalho et al. 2017; Rathi 2016).

80% of patients have chorioretinal involvement, but the majority of these patients do not have visual symptoms (de Melo Marques et al. 2018; Khairallah et al. 2004). Ocular features include retinitis, mild vitritis, and vascular sheathing. The retinitis presents as small white lesions resembling cotton wool spots. These lesions vary in number and size.

Diagnosis is mainly by clinical history and examination, confirmed with immunofluorescence for the rickettsial antigens (Abroug et al. 2014).

Oral doxycycline is used to treat rickettsioses in adults and macrolides such as azithromycin can be used in children. Systemic corticosteroids may be used in severe visual threatening cases (de Melo Marques et al. 2018). Visual prognosis for rickettsiosis is good with appropriate treatment, with little retinal scarring remaining after resolution.

Viral

Acute Retinal Necrosis

Acute retinal necrosis (ARN) was first described in 1971 by Urayama et al. as a rare acute unilateral panuveitis associated with pan-arteritis and subsequent progression to diffuse necrotizing retinitis (Urayama 1971).

Varicella zoster virus (VZV) is known be the main causative agent in around half of the cases reported; followed by herpes simplex virus (HSV) and CMV in adults (Fig. 9.7) (Wong et al. 2010; Ganatra et al. 2000).

Herpes simplex virus type 2 (HSV-2) is the most frequent cause of ARN in younger patients (Van Gelder et al. 2001). HSV-2-mediated ARN may reflect the reactivation of a perinatally-acquired infection, following exposure in the maternal birth canal; and remains latent in the CNS, only to reactivate later, causing ARN (Grose 2012; Silva et al. 2013). ARN predominantly affects immunocompetent individuals, including children, although it has been reported in immunocompromised individuals (Kim et al. 2013; Schoenberger et al. 2017). It is important to note retinal necrosis developed in immunocompromised patients is more likely to present with progressive outer retinal necrosis (PORN) (Fig. 9.8), in which the cluster of differentiation 4 (CD4) count is low and therefore incapable to generate an inflammatory response.

HSV-2 mediated ARN is mostly unilateral, with bilateral disease occurring in less than 10% of cases; but without treatment, 70% of have been shown to progress to bilateral (Schoenberger et al. 2017; Muthiah et al. 2007). Patients present with acute visual loss, photophobia, floaters, and pain.

Foci of retinal necrosis starts at the peripheral retina, and spreads circumferentially toward the posterior pole, progressing rapidly in the absence of treatment. It is characterized by severe vitritis, with retinitis and retinal necrosis (Holland 1994) (See Table 9.2).

Early diagnosis of ARN can be challenging and when it is not obvious clinically, sampling of intraocular fluids for PCR is imperative. Aqueous biopsy carries relatively low risk and high yield.

Retinal holes or tears may develop due to retinal necrosis-induced thinning. These typically appear at the junction of normal and affected retina. Together with subsequent vitreous organization and resultant traction, this leads to rhegmatogenous and/or tractional retinal detachment. The risk of retinal detachment in ARN is 44–75%; which can reduce to 14% with prophylactic vitrectomy (Clarkson et al. 1984; Risseeuw et al. 2019).

The visual prognosis of ARN is generally poor, as these patients often have advanced disease by the time antiviral therapy is initiated (Iwahashi-Shima et al. 2013; Ishida et al. 2009; Watanabe et al. 2011). A greater extent of retinitis at the onset, and delay in presentation, predict a poorer visual outcome due to retinal detachment, retinal ischemia, and optic atrophy (Hillenkamp et al. 2009; Meghpara et al. 2010; Roy et al. 2014).

Early and aggressive treatment is the cornerstone of ARN management (Fig. 9.9). The primary aim is rapid

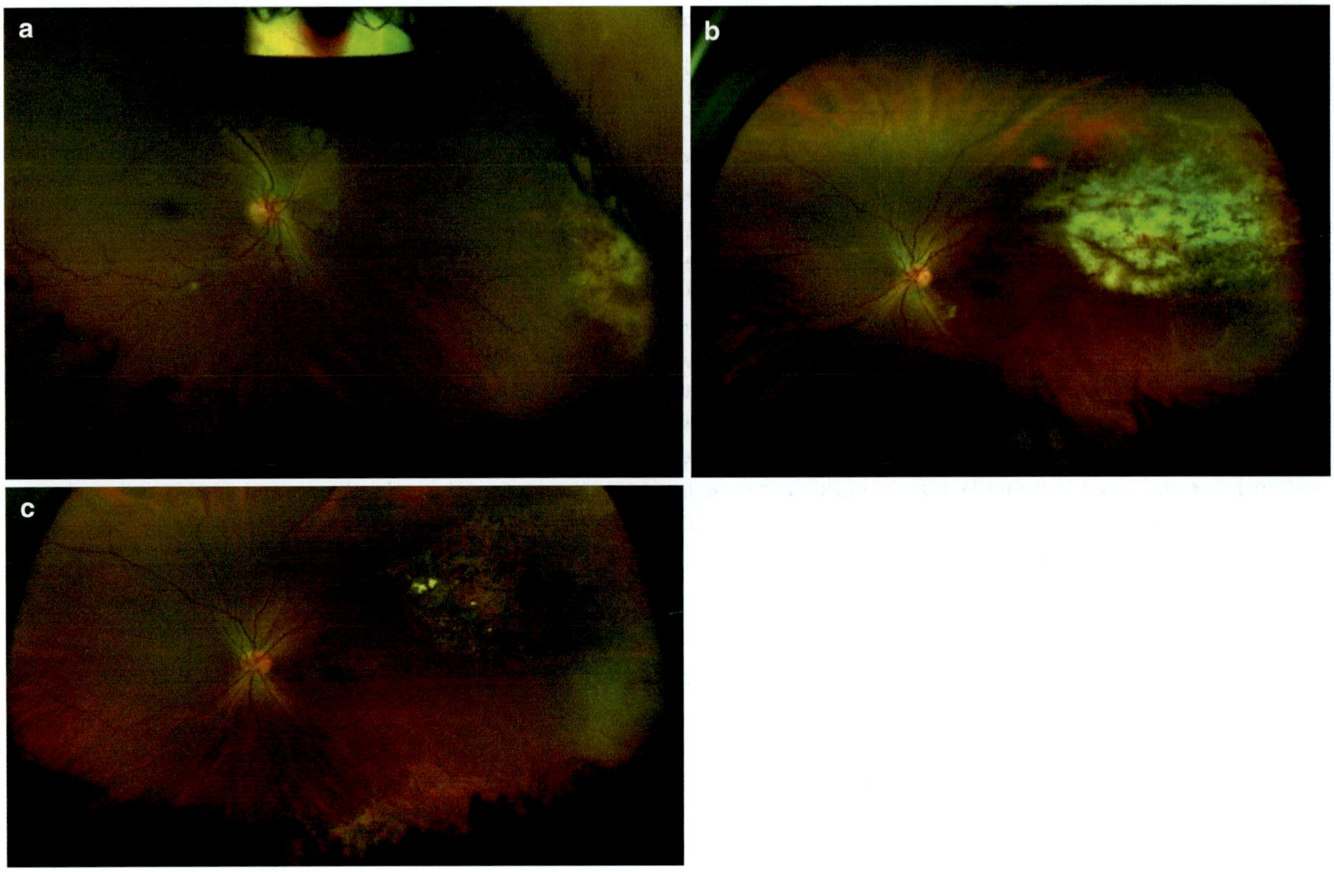

Fig. 9.7 (**a**) and (**b**) A 13 years old with a 5-week history of feeling unwell, blurry vision, and increasing floaters, 6 months after a CMV mismatched heart transplant for a congenital cardiac anomaly. The child was asplenic and on tacrolimus, azathioprine, and prednisolone to prevent rejection of the transplanted heart. The child was found to have bilateral retinitis shown in this optos fundus image of the right (**a**) and left (**b**) eye demonstrating right peripheral nasal half retinitis and left superior temporal retinal necrosis extended inferiorly. He had a high CMV titre postoperatively of 996,448 IU/ml (1,713,890 copies/ml $\log^6$) and CMV associated hepatitis. (**c**) Optos fundus image of the left eye showing complete resolution of ARN after intravenous acyclovir with pigmented retinal atrophy

recovery and prevention of fellow eye involvement. The therapeutic regimen consists of high-dose intravenous acyclovir until a response is detectable, usually within 10 days, followed by prolonged maintenance oral antiviral agents, e.g. acyclovir, valacyclovir, ganciclovir, valganciclovir, or famciclovir. Combined systemic and intravitreal therapy with ganciclovir or Foscarnet has shown promising outcomes (Flaxel et al. 2013; Chen et al. 2016). Poor response to acyclovir may be due to CMV or acyclovir-resistant HSV or VZV.

In spite of effective antiviral therapy, vitritis and vitreous organization will continue to progress due to the inflammatory reaction. Corticosteroids can help to reduce intraocular inflammation and clear the vitreous opacification in ARN. The use of corticosteroids in ARN, however, remains controversial. Some believe that it may facilitate viral replication and worsen the underlying infection in the affected eye, or trigger an infection in the unaffected contralateral eye; while others believe that the outcomes can be favourable (Pikkel and Pikkel 2014).

The value of confluent laser photocoagulation used as prophylaxis for retinal detachment in ARN is also debatable. Laser applied posterior to the areas of active retinitis can create a barrier posterior to where retinal holes are likely to develop (Sternberg Jr et al. 1988), although the usefulness in reducing the risks of retinal detachment is not universally agreed (Roy et al. 2014). Laser photocoagulation is more likely to succeed in eyes with mild ARN, less vitritis, and a relatively clear media. These eyes inherently have a better visual prognosis compared to eyes with more severe disease, where the vitritis precludes the application of laser, and often it is impossible to differentiate between the affected and uninvolved retina due to ill-defined borders.

Lastly, the outcomes from prophylactic vitrectomy remain unsatisfactory and has a high re-operative rate.

Fungal

Fungi are commonly divided into yeasts and moulds, of particular note in retinal inflammation is *Candida*. Fungi are everywhere in nature, but very few cause issues in humans,

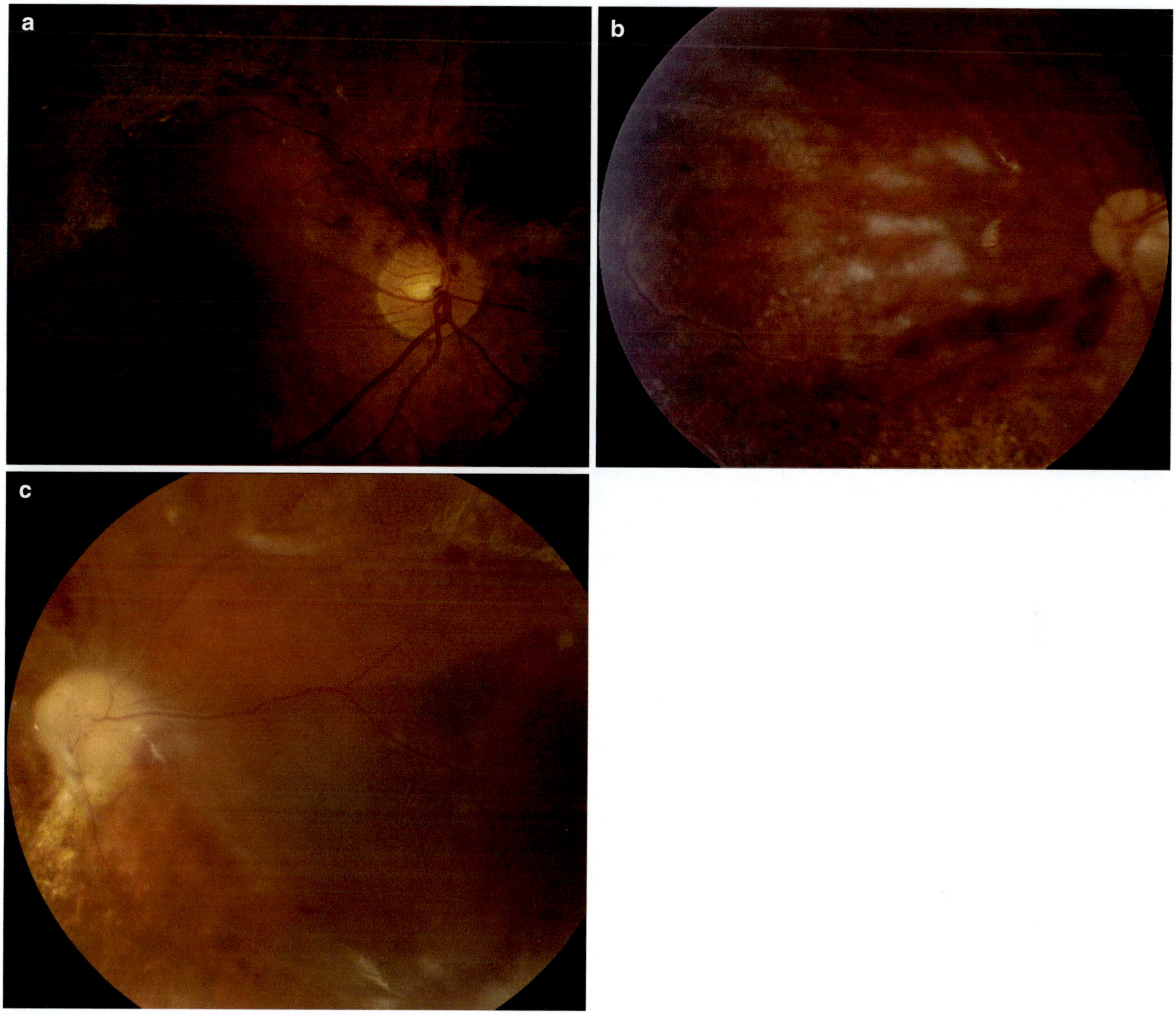

Fig. 9.8 (**a**) and (**b**) A colour fundus image of the right posterior pole and left nasal retina from a young child, presenting with bilateral circumferential necrotizing retinitis without significant intraocular inflammation, while severely immunosuppressed during chemotherapy for relapsed acute lymphoblastic leukaemia. PCR confirmed this to be CMV at vitreous biopsy. (**c**) A colour fundus image of the left eye. Despite high-dose intravenous antivirals and weekly intravitreal Foscarnet (2.4 mg/0.1 ml), the retinitis continued to deteriorate, resulting in occlusive vasculopathy and optic atrophy

Table 9.2 Diagnostic criteria of ARN

Diagnostic criteria on late ocular features in ARN American Uveitis Society (Holland 1994)
One or more discrete foci of peripheral retinal necrosis outside of the major vascular arcades
Circumferential spread
Occlusive vasculopathy with arteriolar involvement
A prominent vitreous or anterior chamber inflammatory reaction
Rapid disease progression in the absence of antiviral therapy

the most common fungal infection is *Candida*. Ocular fungal infection is quite rare but can be sight threatening in the infected eye. Ocular fungal infection can be endogenous or exogenous. Endogenous infection is spread through the bloodstream during systemic infection, the fungi anchor in the choroid or retina, resulting in choroiditis, chorioretinitis, or retinitis (Parke et al. 1982). Risk factors for endogenous infection include systemic corticosteroid or antibiotic treat-

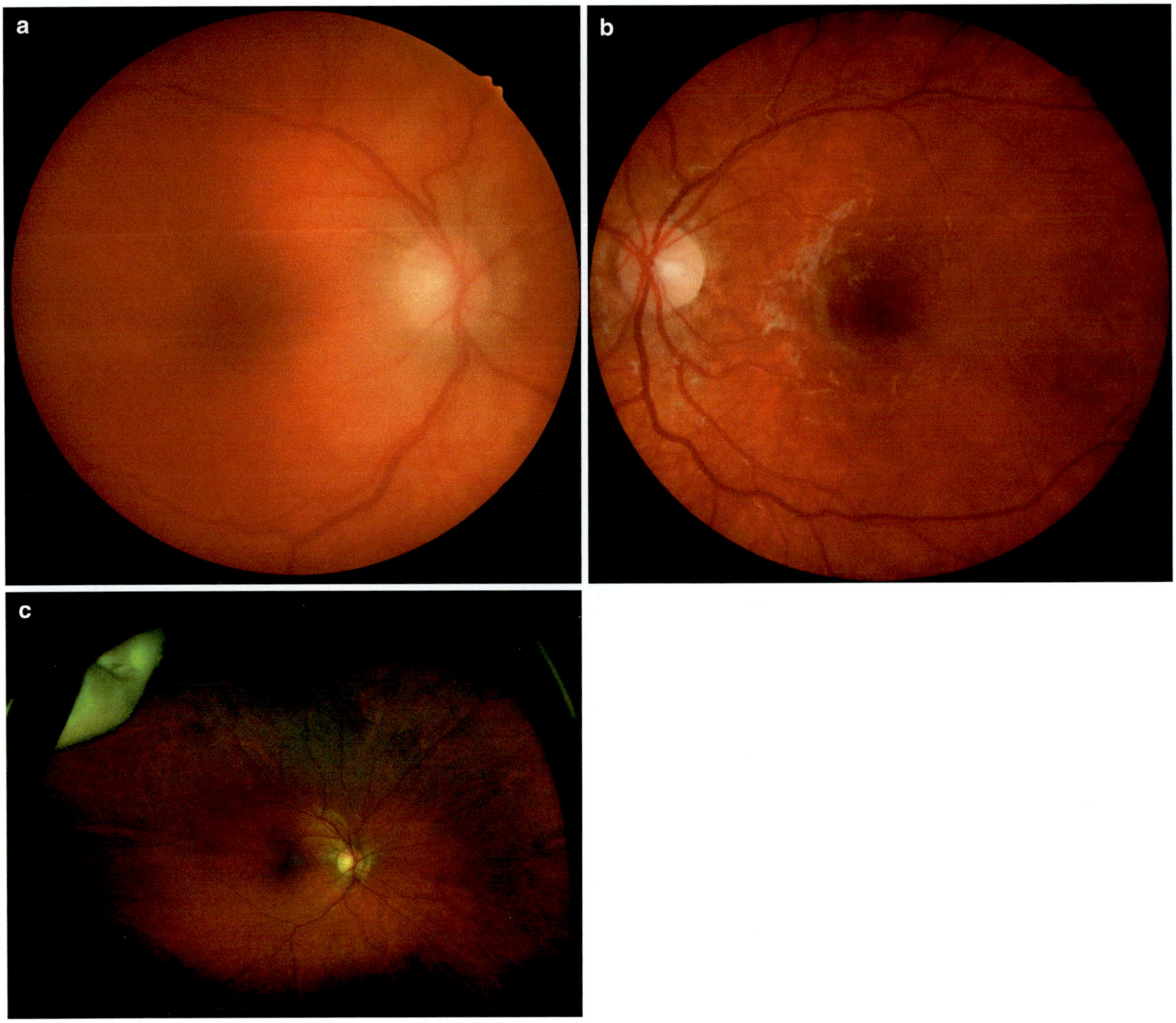

Fig. 9.9 (**a**) and (**b**) Colour fundus photo of the right and left eye. A 4-year-old was on maintenance chemotherapy for precursor B cell acute lymphoblastic leukaemia, which included weekly oral methotrexate, monthly intravenous vincristine, oral dexamethasone, and 3 monthly intrathecal methotrexate. He was admitted for intravenous acyclovir within 48 h of developing <6 nonspecific non-vesicular papules in multiple dermatomes, treated as disseminated VZV after skin swab confirmed VZV DNA on PCR. At the time of admission, the mother noticed a mildly red right eye with no pain. Ocular assessments found reduced vision at 6/38 in the right eye due to right dense vitritis with no retinitis. (**c**) Optos fundus image of the right eye after aqueous biopsy confirming VZV on PCR and no malignant cells. The vision improved to 6/6, after intravitreal Foscarnet and intravenous acyclovir. Active antiviral treatment had stopped the development of retinitis in this mildly immunocompromised child

ment, severe sepsis or septic shock, total parenteral nutrition, surgery, and immunosuppression (Fig. 9.10) (Eggimann and Pittet 2014; Narendran et al. 2008). Exogenous infections are often due to ocular trauma or surgery.

Candida

The yeast *Candida* is part of the normal flora of humans, residing in the respiratory, gastrointestinal, and genital tract. They are a commensal organism but can become pathogenic and potential fatal if the host is immunocompromised (Edwards Jr 1995). Vulvovaginitis, skin infection, and nail infection are the most common manifestations of candidiasis, with ocular involvement being relatively rare and on the decrease with an incidence of less than 2% for patients infected with *Candida* (Shah et al. 2008; Griffin et al. 1973). Around 3% of children with candidemia have been shown to

Fig. 9.10 A colour fundus image from a 13-year-old child's right retina, presenting with pain during chemotherapy for acute lymphoblastic leukaemia. Culture of skin from the foot showed fusarium leading to endogenous endophthalmitis and a rapidly progressive retinitis at the inferior temporal quadrant

have intraocular involvement, although there is very little research on the epidemiology and clinical characteristics in children (Fierro et al. 2013).

Candida albicans is the most common ocular *Candida* infection, followed by *Candida parapsilosis* and *Candida tropicalis* (Edwards Jr et al. 1974). Ocular infections are usually caused by haematogenous spread into the choroid and retina through small capillaries. The fungi then proliferate, causing focal inflammation and local abscess formation (Fig. 9.11). Spread to the vitreous body may cause frank endophthalmitis and retinal detachment. Common presenting symptoms include blurry vision, pain, photophobia, and red eyes (Shah et al. 2008; Griffin et al. 1973).

Chorioretinitis in Candida presents as single or multifocal deep white/yellow lesions. As the disease progresses, inflammation spreads into the vitreous forming cotton ball opacities connected by "strings of pearls". Variable anterior chamber reactions can be observed with an occasional hypopyon. Bilateral involvement is common, although the disease is usually asymmetric (Donahue et al. 1994). Lens abscess, vitreous abscess, Roth spots, and intraretinal haemorrhage can all be other signs of intraocular candidiasis.

Intraocular candidiasis can present silently, so it is recommended all patients with candidemia have ophthalmic examination. Prompt use of antifungals in those with candidemia has been shown to reduce the incidence and severity of intraocular infection (Scherer and Lee 1997).

Diagnosis can be assisted by microscopic examination of the fungus or growth in samples. Growth from a blood sample is highly suggestive of candidemia. Vitreous fluid collection by pars plana vitrectomy can isolate the fungus for culture, but sensitivity has been shown to be less than 50% (Martinez-Vaquez et al. 1998). PCR has been shown to be promising in diagnosis, with a higher sensitivity than culture and provides the benefit of allowing species identification (Anand et al. 2001; Jaeger et al. 2000; Okhravi et al. 1998).

Intravenous antifungals with agents such as amphotericin B, fluconazole, and caspofungin are used for systemic candidiasis. Intravitreal antifungals (Fig. 9.11c) are the standard approach for ocular manifestations combined with pars plana vitrectomy (Khan et al. 2007).

Parasites

Toxoplasmosis

Ocular toxoplasmosis is a known cause of infectious retinitis globally. Toxoplasmosis infects approximately one-third of the world's population, but prevalence varies depending on dietary habit, hygiene, and climate (Subauste et al. 2011). The incidences have been reported between 0.8 per 100,000 per year in British-born individuals versus 77 per 100,000 per year for those born in west Africa (Gilbert et al. 1995). Both genders have been shown to be equally affected (Garza-Leon and Arellanes 2012). Toxoplasmosis is a zoonotic infection caused by *Toxoplasma gondii* (*T. Gondii*), an obligate intracellular parasite. Cats are the definitive primary host of *T. Gondii* and excrete oocysts in their faeces which then infect intermediate hosts such as humans or other warm-blooded animals. Toxoplasmosis infection may be congenital (transplacental) or acquired by ingesting tissue cysts present in contaminated material.

Tachyzoites and tissue cysts are present in the intermediate hosts, while oocysts are produced only in cat intestines. The intermediate host ingests the cyst and produces tachyzoites which in turn causes disease. Lysis of the host cell results in the release and spread of tachyzoites and can manifest as necrotizing retinitis. Bradyzoites are the quiescent form of *T. Gondii* and remain dormant in tissue cysts; but when ruptured, can reactivate retinitis (Silveira et al. 2011).

Chorioretinal atrophy with hyperpigmentation around the borders is indicative of inactive disease (Fig. 9.12), with 71.4% of paediatric patients reported to have inactive disease (Garza-Leon and Arellanes 2012). Lesions involving the peripheral retina have little impact on quality of life and visual function (Peyron et al. 2011).

Most active disease can present with acute symptoms such as visual loss, floaters, or painful red eye, although more commonly it can be asymptomatic and found incidentally in children with strabismus, poor vision, or phthisis bulbi (Garza-Leon and Arellanes 2012; Stanford et al. 2006).

During an active episode, panuveitis is the most common manifestation (50%) (Garza-Leon and Arellanes 2012; Stanford et al. 2006; Bosch-Driessen et al. 2002), there is focal necrotizing retinitis of the inner retina, as well as a sec-

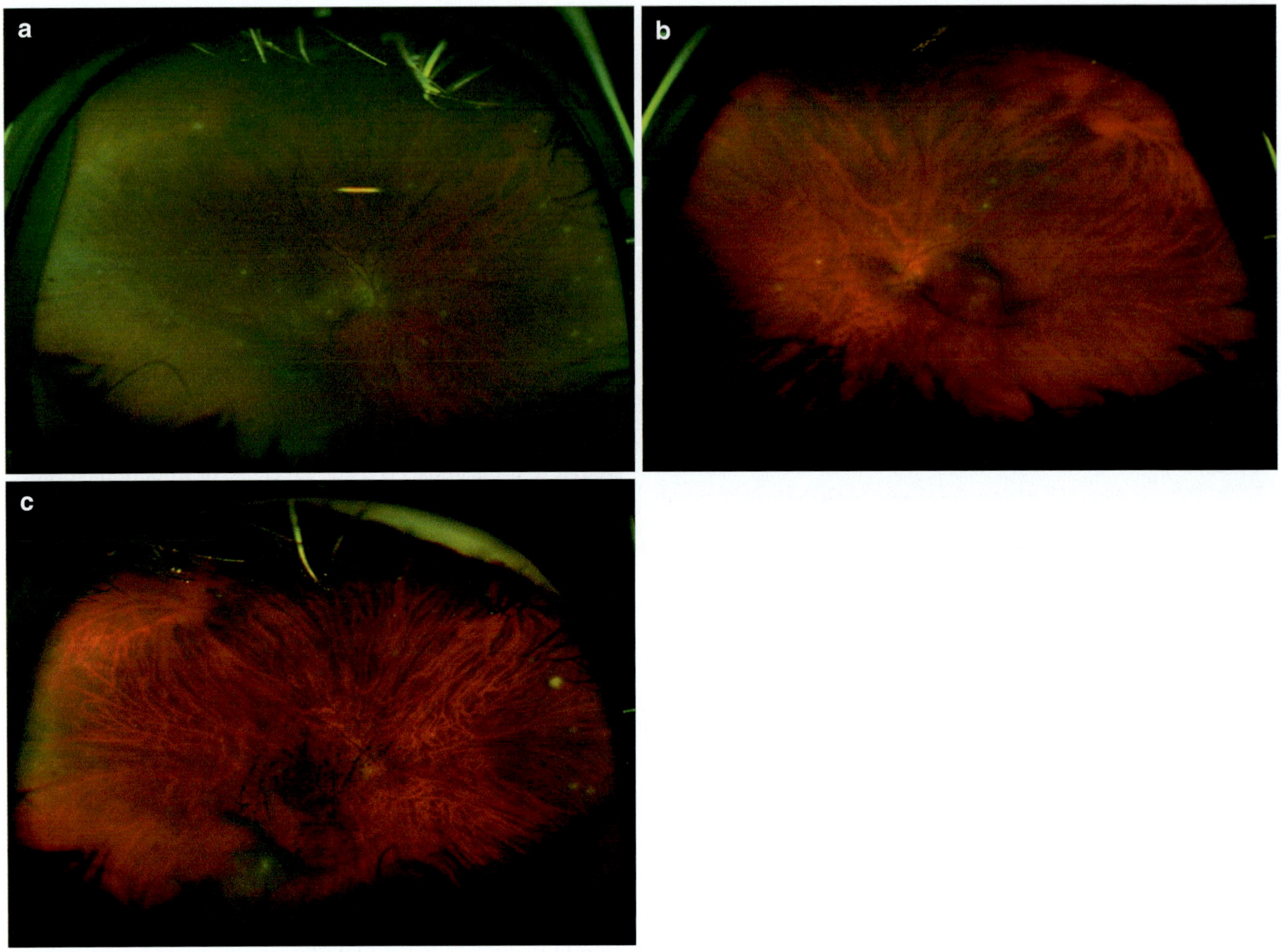

Fig. 9.11 (**a**) and (**b**) Optos image of the right and left eye from a 17-year-old diagnosed with bilateral multifocal chorioretinitis with vitritis; presenting with symptoms of blurred vision, and general unwellness. Candidemia was confirmed in blood culture during systemic workup. The causation was thought to be related to recreational intravenous drug use. (**c**) An optos image of the worse affected right eye from (**a**) showed improvement 1 week after intravitreal amphotericin injection. Pars plana vitrectomy was performed when general health improved, and a visual acuity of 6/6 was retained in both eyes

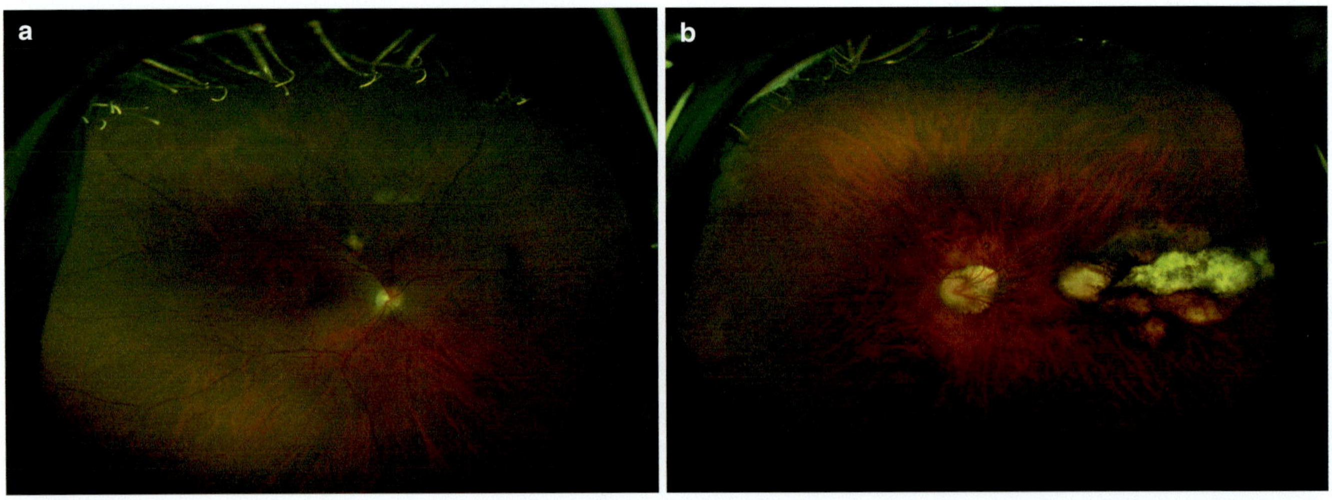

Fig. 9.12 (**a**) and (**b**) An optos fundus image of the right and left eye from a 14-year-old presenting with psychosocially symptomatic left sensory exotropia. Her vision was 6/5 in the right and 6/60 in the left eye due to inactive scars involving the macula

ondary inflammatory response of the choroid, vitreous, and retinal vessels (Nussenblatt and Belfort 1994; Rothova 1993; Holland 2000). The active lesion is typically fluffy yellowish-white in colour (Garza-Leon and Arellanes 2012). Reactivation of the infection is characterized by new active lesions adjacent to old atrophic scars (Nussenblatt and Belfort 1994; Holland 2004). Marked vitritis overlying active retinal lesions is classically described as a 'headlight in the fog' appearance.

Children with active ocular toxoplasmosis have been shown to have a higher frequency (56.2%) of retinal vasculitis compared to patients of all ages (24%) (Garza-Leon and Arellanes 2012; De-la-Torre et al. 2009). Optic nerve involvement may be observed as anterior neuritis or papillitis, or as neuroretinitis but is relatively rare (Garza-Leon and Arellanes 2012; Roach et al. 1985; Eckert et al. 2007).

Ocular complications include retinal breaks (5%), retinal detachment (6%), choroidal neovascularisation and cataract (11.6%) (Bosch-Driessen et al. 2000; Arun et al. 2007). Poor visual outcomes in ocular toxoplasmosis are usually secondary to macular involvement.

Diagnosis of ocular toxoplasmosis is always clinical, serological tests have limited use. Due to the high seropositivity and lifelong persistence of IgG antibodies (Roberts et al. 2001); anti-*T. gondii* IgG are only useful in excluding the diagnosis if they are absent. Real-time PCR can be used when tissue biopsy is obtained.

Acute toxoplasma chorioretinitis tends to be self-limiting. The goal of treatment is to arrest multiplication of the protozoa during the active phase of inflammation, thereby minimizing the duration and intensity of intraocular inflammation that can lead to irreversible damage to the macula and optic nerve. The most commonly used treatment regime for ocular toxoplasmosis is a combination of pyrimethamine and sulfadiazine, which inhibit DNA synthesis. Alternative regimes include trimethoprim/sulfamethoxazole, clindamycin, and azithromycin. However, none of these treatments have been shown to penetrate the tissue cysts, therefore do not eradicate the bradyzoites within (Stanford and Gilbert 2009). As the tissue cysts remain in the retina there is a potential lifelong risk of recurrence.

Toxocariasis

Toxocariasis is a roundworm parasitic disease found globally, humans acquire toxocariasis by ingestion of the larvae of *Toxocara* from either dog (*Toxocara canis*) or cat (*Toxocara cati*); toxocariasis is considered a poverty-related neglect disease. Transmission is faecal–oral from accidental ingestion of contaminated material, e.g. food, water, or soil (Yoshikawa et al. 2008; Yamada et al. 2006; Manini et al. 2012). The global prevalence is reported as 11.1% (Rostami et al. 2020a) in dogs and 17.0% (Rostami et al. 2020b) in cats; and owners are more likely to be infected (Won et al. 2008; Fisher 2003; Macpherson 2013). However, human prevalences have been less widely researched, reports range from 8% in the Eastern Mediterranean to 38% in Africa (Rostami et al. 2020b).

Ingested larvae migrate from the small intestine into the portal circulation and then distribute to various organs, such as lungs, liver, muscle, brain, and eyes. The larvae can migrate for an extended period of time or become immobile and produce a vigorous eosinophilic granulomatous inflammation, a foreign body response. The older inactive lesions consist of epithelioid cells, with the larva often disintegrated and unrecognizable (Kayes and Oaks 1978).

Toxocariasis may be generalized (visceral larva migrans) or ocular (ocular larva migrans). Children account for the majority of active disease with the generalized form often being self-limiting and subclinical, but rarely it can be fatal due to cardiac, pulmonary, hepatic, or CNS involvement (Desai et al. 2020; Almatary and Bakir 2016).

Wilder first described intraocular larvae infection in 1950 (Wilder 1950). The larva has a diameter of 15–21 μm (Ash 2007), and is trapped in retinal capillaries as they narrow. Therefore, lesions are typically located in the peripheral retina and to a lesser extent in the posterior pole, very occasionally they affect the optic nerve. It is unilateral in 90% of cases (Chieffi et al. 2009; Rubinsky-Elefant et al. 2010).

The active retinal lesion is typically poorly defined with a profound cellular infiltrate, extending into the vitreous, and can cause massive tractional band and retinal folds. Ciliary body inflammation can mimic snowbanking in pars planitis. Children with *Toxocara*-related chronic endophthalmitis are often younger and asymptomatic; they can present with leukocoria, strabismus, or visual loss. Key clinical features include intense vitritis, ill-defined retinitis with granuloma, and low-to-moderate anterior uveitis, although hypopyon has been reported (Ahn et al. 2014a).

Ocular toxocariasis presents at a young age with dense vitritis and retinal granuloma, this can pose a diagnostic dilemma and resemble endophytic retinoblastoma; 7% of pseudoretinoblastoma can be attributed to *Toxocara* (Shields et al. 2013). Retinal detachment has been reported as 18–65% (Kwon et al. 2011; Liu et al. 2016), with some cases of proliferative vitreoretinopathy and neovascularisation. Tractional retinal or ciliary body detachment with hypotony can lead to phthisis bulbi and severe visual loss. Persisting posterior retinal fold, macular oedema, maculopathy, and epiretinal membrane can also lead to poor visual outcomes (Sahu et al. 2018).

Ocular toxocariasis is usually a clinical diagnosis after careful history and examination with B-scan ultrasonography and ultra-wide-field retinal imaging. Diagnostic vitrectomy, division of retinal traction, intraoperative examination, and sampling can be useful in cases where it is not possible to achieve a fundal view.

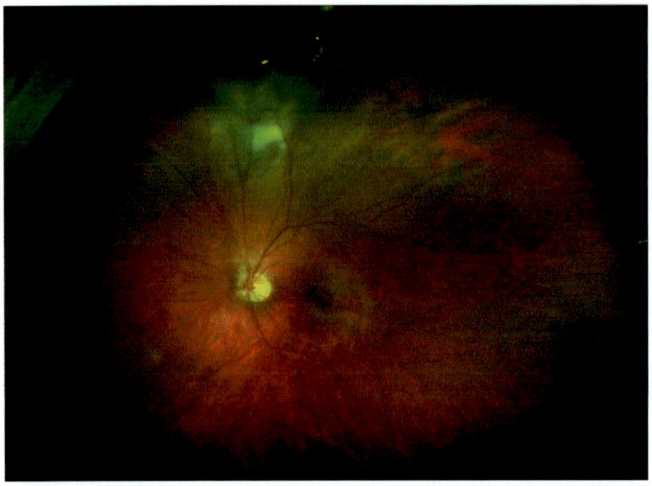

Fig. 9.13 An optos fundus image of the left eye from a 9-year-old presenting with left uniocular red eye and found to have profound sight loss with vision of hand movement, dense vitritis and no fundal view. He underwent B-scan assessment followed by diagnostic pars plana vitrectomy and found to have retinitis superiorly with choroidal granuloma and retinal folds. PCR confirmed toxocara

The standard diagnostic test for *Toxocara* is ELISA which uses the crude antigen of the larvae and is highly sensitive and specific. Serum immunoglobulin levels can play a supportive role in the diagnosis, with 69.6% of ocular toxocariasis reported to have elevated IgE levels. Systemic toxocariasis usually has eosinophilia, but is often absent in the ocular form (Ahn et al. 2014b).

The treatment strategy depends on the degree of intraocular inflammation and vitreoretinal complications. The primary aim of treatment is to minimize inflammation and prevent the formation of membranes or tractional bands. The role of antihelmintics remains uncertain in ocular toxocariasis, combined treatment with albendazole and corticosteroids appears to be effective in reducing the recurrence of intraocular inflammation (Ahn et al. 2014a).

Surgery is indicated for complications such as persistent vitreous opacification, retinal detachment, epiretinal membrane with vitreomacular traction, and recurrent inflammation. Timely vitrectomy could rescue vision but prognosis remains unfavourable (Zhang et al. 2020) (Fig. 9.13).

Non-infectious Entities

Vogt–Koyanagi–Harada Syndrome

Vogt–Koyanagi–Harada (VKH) disease was first described in 1906 by Vogt as a uveitis with poliosis; in 1929 Koyanagi reported bilateral uveitis with poliosis, vitiligo, dysacousia, and alopecia; in 1926 Harada reported a disease characterized by serous retinal detachment and cerebrospinal fluid abnormalities as a uveitic entity. Subsequent studies suggested Vogt, Koyanagi, and Harada were the same syndrome but at different stages. In 2007 Yang revealed that Harada disease is an early manifestation, whereas Vogt-Koyanagi syndrome is the recurrent stage, hence solidifying the syndrome as a whole (Yang et al. 2007).

Table 9.3 Genes associated with VKH (Hou et al. 2014; Islam et al. 1994)

HLA associated with VKH	Single-nucleotide polymorphisms associated with VKH (non-HLA)	Copy number variations of immune-related genes associated with VKH
DR4	CTLA-4	C4
DRw53	SUMO4	C3
DQw3	PTPN22	IL-17F
B54	IFN-γ	IL-23A
DQ4	IL-17	FAS
DR1	IL-12B	
DRB1*0405	TLR9	
DQA1*0301	TNIP1	
DQB1*0401	NLRP1	
	OPN	
	miR-146a	

VKH predominantly affects pigmented races, especially in Sino-Asians, South and Central Americans, native Americans, and Middle-Easterners. It is less common in European and North American populations (Du et al. 2016).

VKH is a chronic multisystem autoimmune disease that targets the meninges, inner ear, and melanin-containing cells. The exact pathogenesis of VKH remains uncertain, and is proposed to be a combination of a T-cell mediated autoimmune reaction against melanin or melanin-related antigens, triggered by an infection in the genetically susceptible individual (Eggimann and Pittet 2014). Various class II human leukocyte antigens (HLA) have been linked (e.g. HLA-DR4) in the Japanese population, HLA-DRB1*0405, DQA1*0301, and DQB1*0401 in the Chinese cohorts (Hou et al. 2014; Islam et al. 1994). Other genetic associations are listed below (See Table 9.3).

VKH is relatively uncommon in children; only 3–13.4% of patients with VKH are under 16 years old, with the youngest reported case being 3 years old (Chen et al. 2016; Pikkel and Pikkel 2014; Sternberg Jr et al. 1988).

VKH may present with ocular (bilateral panuveitis), neurological (meningitis, lymphocytic pleocytosis), integumentary (vitiligo and poliosis) and/or auditory manifestations (sensorineural hearing loss) (Moorthy et al. 1995; Rajendram et al. 2005; Chi et al. 2007). A classification system is shown below (See Table 9.4).

VKH in children is aggressive with worse ocular complications, e.g. glaucoma and cataract requiring surgery (Tabbara et al. 1998; Ohno et al. 1988). More than 20% of all

Table 9.4 Classification system for the clinical stages of VKH developed by Yang et al. (2007)

Stages	Clinical features
Prodromal stage (about 1 or 2 weeks before uveitis attack)	Headache, fever, meningism, hearing loss, tinnitus, stiffness of neck and back
Posterior uveitis stage (about 2 weeks after uveitis attack)	Chorioretinitis, exudative retinal detachment, optic disc oedema or hyperaemia
Anterior uveal involvement stage (from 2 weeks to 2 months after uveitis attack)	Active posterior uveitis, non-granulomatous anterior uveitis
Recurrent granulomatous anterior uveitis stage (more than 2 months after uveitis attack)	"Sunset glow" fundus, Dalen-Fuchs nodules, recurrent granulomatous, Koeppe and Busacca nodules, ocular complications, e.g. band keratopathy, cataract, glaucoma, subretinal neovascularisation, retinochoroidal atrophy

children were blind in at least one eye at their initial presentation (Reiff 2019).

High-dose corticosteroid should be initiated promptly, followed by slow tapering (Iwahashi et al. 2015; Silpa-archa et al. 2016). However, prolonged use of systemic corticosteroids is particularly problematic in children (Perente et al. 2009) and known to cause growth retardation, Cushing syndrome, hyperglycaemia, adrenal suppression, and increased risk of severe infections. The treatment objective is rapid control of inflammation, and to achieve lifelong remission (Jabs et al. 2000). Early referral to the paediatric rheumatologist for initiation of systemic steroid and/or disease-modifying antirheumatic drug (DMARD) therapy improves visual outcomes (Reiff 2019; Paredes et al. 2006; Andreoli and Foster 2006). Biological therapy can be considered for refractory disease (Vallet et al. 2016; Umran and Shukur 2018).

Sarcoidosis

Sarcoidosis is a chronic multisystem disease characterized by non-caseating granulomatous inflammation (Hunninghake et al. 1999). It most commonly affects young adults, and is very rare in children (Shetty and Gedalia 2008). The estimated incidence of paediatric sarcoidosis was roughly 0.25 per 100,000 per year in one of the largest series by a Danish group, although it is likely underdiagnosed given that affected individuals may be asymptomatic. This same group found males and females to be equally affected amongst children (Hoffmann et al. 2004). The proportion of paediatric uveitis patients with ocular sarcoidosis varies from 2.6% (Engelhard et al. 2015) (United States of America) to 6.1% (Morelle et al. 2019) (France). There is a higher incidence among African Americans (74%) (Shetty and Gedalia 2008; Gedalia et al. 2016). This suggests a genetic predisposition to develop sarcoidosis (Spagnolo and du Bois 2007).

Although no defined cause has been demonstrated (Newman et al. 2004; Rybicki and Iannuzzi 2007), exposure to specific environmental, occupational, or infectious agents (*Mycobacteria tuberculosis* and other atypical mycobacteria (Drake and Newman 2006; Gazouli et al. 2005; Song et al. 2005), *Propionibacterium acnes* (Ishige et al. 1999; Nagata et al. 2017) are thought to trigger an exaggerated cellular immune response (Newman et al. 2004; Rybicki et al. 2001).

The distinct forms of childhood sarcoidosis are:

- *Blau syndrome*, also known as familial juvenile systemic granulomatosis, commonly affects children below the age of 5. It is a rare autosomal dominant granulomatous inflammatory condition, with high penetrance, affecting the eyes, joints, and skin. Blau et al. first described the syndrome in 1985 in 11 members of a family across four generations (Blau 1985; Achille et al. 2016). Blau syndrome is reported to be due to a mutation in nucleotide binding oligomerization domain 2 (NOD2), also called caspase recruitment domain-containing protein 15 (CARD15), in chromosome 16q12. The most common ocular presentation is panuveitis, followed by multifocal chorioretinitis, optic atrophy, and peripapillary nodules. 20% of patients with Blau resulted in moderate to severe visual impairment (Sarens et al. 2018; Latkany et al. 2002).
- *Early-onset childhood sarcoidosis* (EOCS) is rare, present in the first 5 years of life, and is likely to have a sporadic mutation of the NOD2 gene. Its clinical presentation is virtually identical to Blau syndrome, and different from sarcoidosis in older children and adults, with only a minority having lung involvement. EOCS is characterized by the triad of arthritis, dermatitis and uveitis (Touitou and Koné-Paut 2008; Häfner and Vogel 1993; Wouters and Rose 2016). Over 75% of patients with EOCS have uveitis (Gedalia et al. 2016; Hoover et al. 1986), most children have arthritis or a rash prior to presenting to the ophthalmologist, although some may not present with the complete triad or may do so only after years (Rosé et al. 2009; Okafuji et al. 2009; Aróstegui et al. 2007; Bhojwani et al. 2009). Unlike the late-onset form, hilar lymphadenopathy and pulmonary disease are rare in EOCS (Touitou and Koné-Paut 2008; Häfner and Vogel 1993; Hetherington 1982).

The CARD15/NOD2 gene is reported to be linked to the susceptibility of developing Crohn's disease, a granulomatous inflammatory bowel condition. EOCS and Blau syndrome has been reported to present as Crohn's disease (Caso et al. 2015; Ogura et al. 2001; Brunner et al. 2006).

- The other form of paediatric sarcoidosis presents around 8–15 years old (Hetherington 1982). Unlike EOCS, it is

Table 9.5 Clinical signs suggested of ocular sarcoidosis by IWOS criteria (Mochizuki et al. 2019)

Clinical signs suggestive of ocular sarcoidosis
Mutton fat keratic precipitates (large and small) and/or iris nodules at pupillary margin (Koeppe) or in stroma (Busacca)
Trabecular meshwork nodules and/or tent-shaped peripheral anterior synechia.
Snowballs/string of pearls vitreous opacities
Multiple chorioretinal peripheral lesions (active and atrophic)
Nodular and/or segmental periphlebitis (± candlewax drippings) and/or macroaneurysm in an inflamed eye
Optic disc nodule(s)/granuloma(s) and/or solitary choroidal nodule
Bilaterality (assessed by clinical examination or investigational tests showing subclinical inflammation)

Table 9.6 Clinical signs suggestive of systemic sarcoidosis by IWOS criteria (Mochizuki et al. 2019)

Clinical signs suggestive of systemic sarcoidosis
Bilateral hilar lymphadenopathy (BHL) by chest X-ray and/or chest computed CT scan.
Negative tuberculin test or interferon-gamma releasing assays.
Elevated serum ACE.
Elevated serum lysozyme.
Elevated CD4/CD8 ratio (>3.5) in bronchoalveolar lavage fluid.
Abnormal accumulation of gallium-67 scintigraphy or 18F-fluorodeoxyglucose positron emission tomography imaging.
Lymphopenia.
Parenchymal lung changes consistent with sarcoidosis, as determined by pulmonologists or radiologists.

not linked to NOD2 mutations (Cimaz and Ansell 2002). Uveitis and arthropathy are less frequent manifestations; but similar to adult sarcoidosis, with multisystem disease (Shetty and Gedalia 2008; Lindsley and Petty 2000; Pattishall and Kendig Jr 1996). Ocular manifestations, such as multifocal chorioretinitis, periphlebitis, and papillitis, are more frequently reported in children than in adults (Hetherington 1982; Pattishall and Kendig Jr 1996; Milman and Selroos 1990), affecting up to 80% (Gedalia et al. 2016). Conjunctival granulomas (Hoover et al. 1986) and dacryoadenitis may also be present (Gedalia et al. 2016) (See Table 9.5).

The definitive diagnosis of sarcoidosis is made when compatible clinical findings and histopathological evidence of non-caseating granulomas in affected organs (e.g. skin, conjunctiva) while other granulomatous disorders (including TB) are excluded (See Table 9.6).

Serum levels of angiotensin-converting enzyme (ACE) and lysozyme, which measure macrophage products produced by sarcoid granulomas, are often elevated. However, as serum ACE is commonly elevated in children, it cannot be used for the diagnosis of childhood sarcoidosis. Raised serum lysozyme has better specificity and positive predictive values for sarcoidosis than raised serum ACE levels (Kawaguchi et al. 2007).

The course and prognosis of childhood sarcoidosis may correlate with the mode of onset and the extent of the disease. Children with EOCS have a guarded prognosis with the likelihood of a chronic progressive course; 80–100% of these children develop residua of uveitis, polyarthritis, and other organ involvement (Hunninghake et al. 1999; Fauroux and Clément 2005; Fink and Cimaz 1997).

Behçet Disease

Behçet disease (BD) is a relapsing multifactorial systemic inflammatory disorder of unknown etiology first described by Hulusi Behçet et al. (1937). However, the earliest description dates back to around 400 BC in the Epidemics book III of Hippocrates of Kos (Feigenbaum 1956). Behçet described the association of oral and genital aphthous ulcers alongside intraocular inflammation that forms the classic triad of BD.

In addition to the classic triad, necrotizing vasculitis can also affect the skin, joints, mucosal tissues, blood vessels, lungs, CNS, and gastrointestinal system (Gül 2015). The revised International Chapel Hill Consensus Conference defines BD as a "variable vessel vasculitis" meaning it can affect vessels of any size or type (arteries, veins, capillaries) (Jennette et al. 2013).

BD has the highest prevalence rates reported in Jordan (66/10,000) and Turkey (42/10,000), it is highly prevalent throughout the Eastern Mediterranean, Middle East, and North Africa, typically along the traditional route of the silk road; while less commonly seen in Northern Europe and the United Kingdom (UK) (0.6/10,000). The prevalence of BD correlates with the frequency of HLA-B51 in the healthy population. The further east along the silk road, the higher the occurrence of HLA-B51, and thus the higher the prevalence of BD (Ohno et al. 1982; Azizlerli et al. 2003; Madanat et al. 2017). Male to female ratio of BD varies depending on country with the UK having ratios reported at 0.6:1 compared with a ratio of 5.37:1 reported in Egypt (Davatchi et al. 2012). Uveitis, vascular, and neurological involvement is more common in males with BD (Kural-Seyahi et al. 2003; Zouboulis 1999). BD usually develops in the third decade, with younger patients having a more severe disease course. Approximately 50–80% of BD patients developed ocular symptoms, with roughly one-third of these developing retinal vasculitis (Ohno et al. 1982; Azizlerli et al. 2003; Madanat et al. 2017; Davatchi et al. 2016).

The etiology and pathogenesis of BD is not clear currently, although a strong association between HLA-B51 and BD has been established since 1973 by Ohno et al. (1982). Multiple subsequent studies have shown the link between

Table 9.7 HLA genetic associations with Behçet disease (Ombrello et al. 2014)

HLA alleles with an increased risk	HLA alleles with a protective effect and decreased risk
HLA-B15	HLA-B49
HLA-B27	HLA-A03
HLA-B57	
HLA-A26	

Table 9.8 Non-HLA genetic associations with an increased risk of developing Behçet disease (Kirino et al. 2013a, b; Remmers et al. 2010; Takeuchi et al. 2017)

Immune response genes	Sensing and danger signals genes
IL-10	ERAP1
IL23-R	MEFV
IL-1α/IL-1β	TLR4
CCR1	NOD2
STAT4	LACCI
IRF8	FUT2
CEBPB-PTPN1	
RIPK2	
ADO-EGR2	

HLA-B51 and BD in the following years showing that around 40–80% of BD patients have HLA-B51, compared to 10–30% in control populations (Chang et al. 2001; Choukri et al. 2001; Kilmartin et al. 1997; Chung et al. 1987; Boura et al. 2007; Houman et al. 2007). There are weaker associations with other HLA variants as well as other non-HLA gene variants (See Tables 9.7 and 9.8). Pathogenic connections with *Streptococcus sanguinis* and HSV and BD have also been established (Young et al. 1988; Yoshikawa et al. 1998).

Multiple diagnostic criteria have been made for paediatric BD (See Table 9.9).

Ocular BD often starts as unilateral anterior uveitis, but bilateral posterior uveitis occurs in up to 78% of cases, with 60% developing chronic relapsing panuveitis (Tugal-Tutkun et al. 2004). Retinal vasculitis in BD affects both central and peripheral retinal vessels, resulting in retinal haemorrhages and soft exudates (Fig. 9.14). The optic disc may be swollen, and optic neuritis may also be present. Necrotising obliterative vasculitis may result in neovascularisation of the optic disc and/or the peripheral retina, these can lead to retinal detachment and/or vitreous haemorrhage and neovascular glaucoma.

The management aims in BD are to treat acute inflammatory attacks and to prevent future inflammatory attacks; this often involves multiple specialities. High-dose intravenous methylprednisolone is often the most effective therapy in treating hyperacute sight-threatening recurrences of retinal inflammation (Figs. 9.14 and 9.15).

Table 9.9 Paediatric diagnostic criteria for Behçet disease. Three of six clinical features are required to classify a patient as having paediatric Behçet disease (Koné-Paut et al. 2016)

Clinical feature	Description
Recurrent oral aphthosis	At least three attacks/year
Genital ulceration or aphthosis	Typically, with scar
Skin involvement	Necrotic folliculitis, acneiform lesions, erythema nodosum
Ocular involvement	Anterior uveitis, posterior uveitis, retinal vasculitis
Neurological signs	With the exception of isolated headaches
Vascular signs	Venous thrombosis, arterial thrombosis, arterial aneurysm

Long-term uses of systemic steroids alone have its associated side effects and are often not adequate in preventing acute recurrences. Systemic agents used in treating eye inflammation include azathioprine (Yazici et al. 1990; Saadoun et al. 2010), cyclophosphamide (Davatchi et al. 2004), cyclosporin (Özdal et al. 2002), mycophenolate mofetil, biologic therapy e.g. infliximab (anti-tumour necrosis factor α) (Tugal-Tutkun et al. 2005), rituximab (anti-CD20 monoclonal antibody) and anakinra (interleukin-1-6R receptor antagonist).

Idiopathic Retinal Vasculitis, Aneurysms, and Neuroretinitis Syndrome

In 1995 Chang et al. observed a rare ocular pathology seen before in 1973 by Karel et al. and in 1983 by Kincaid and Schatz that developed bilaterally in young healthy female patients with no systemic association; naming it idiopathic retinal vasculitis, aneurysms, and neuroretinitis (IRVAN) syndrome.

There are three main criteria and three minor criteria for diagnosing IRVAN syndrome (Kincaid and Schatz 1983) (See Table 9.10).

Patients are often asymptomatic at presentation despite quite dramatic retinal findings, if left untreated; exudative maculopathy, retinal damage, and neovascular glaucoma can lead to severe visual loss. The presence of multiple aneurysmal dilatations of the retinal and optic nerve head arterioles is one of the characteristic clinical features of IRVAN, these vascular anomalies can measure between 75 and 300 μm in diameter and can be present at or near major branching sites on retinal arterioles. These dilatations may be triangular or "Y" shaped giving the appearance of knots tied in the vasculature (Chang et al. 1995; Yeshurun et al. 2003). IRVAN aneurysms tend to leak, causing lipid depositions extending to the fovea (Fig. 9.16), peripheral capillary nonperfusion (Fig. 9.5) can lead to the development of preretinal neovascularisation and vaso-proliferative complications including

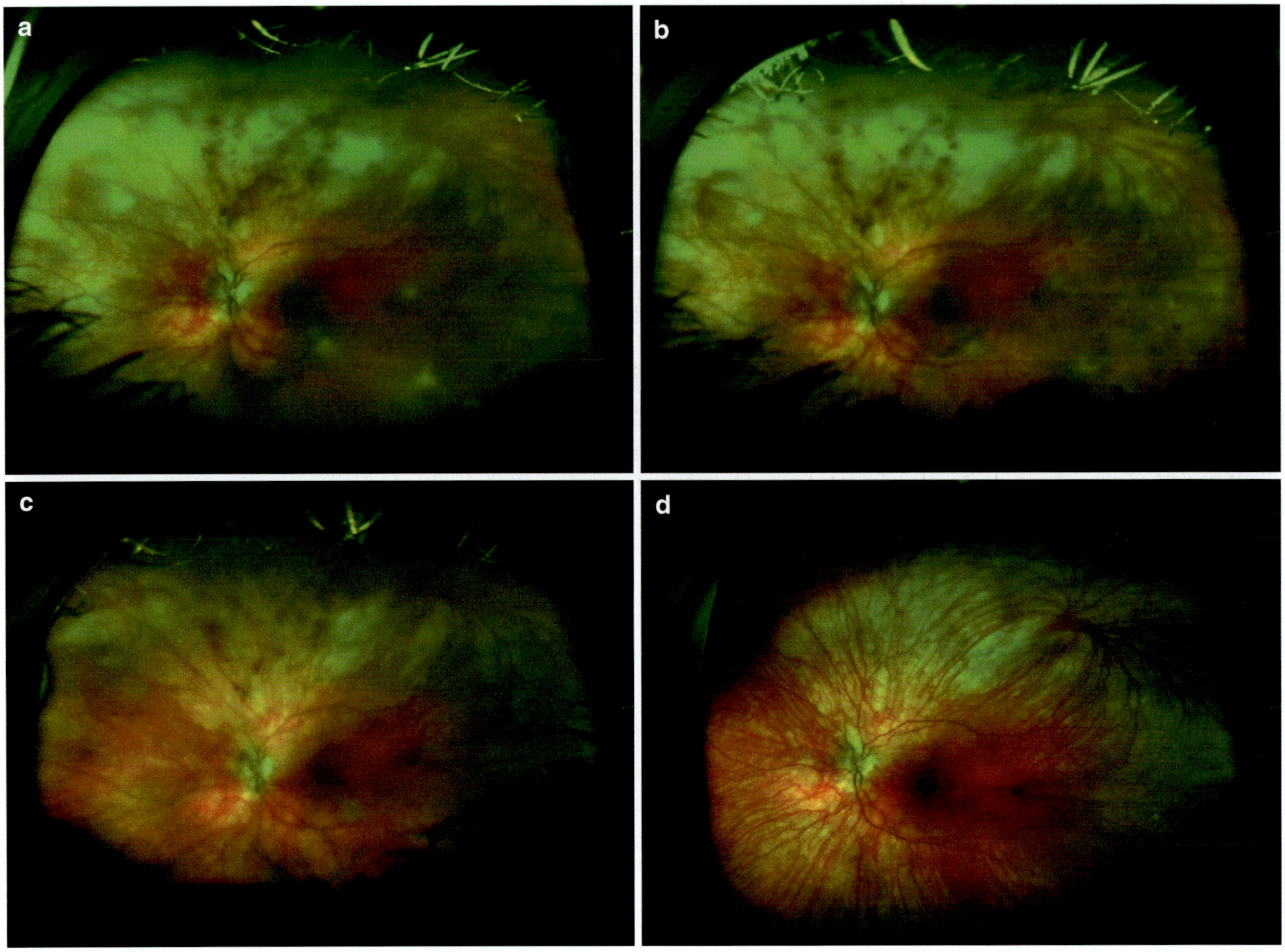

Fig. 9.14 (**a**) An optos fundus image of the left eye during a relapse demonstrating vitritis, multifocal chorioretinitis, superior pseudo-ARN, retinal haemorrhages, and exudation. (**b**) and (**c**) Optos fundus images showing rapid resolution of retinal vasculitis, 1 day and 2 days after intravenous methyl prednisolone. (**d**) Optos fundus images showing complete resolution of retinal vasculitis, 2 weeks later

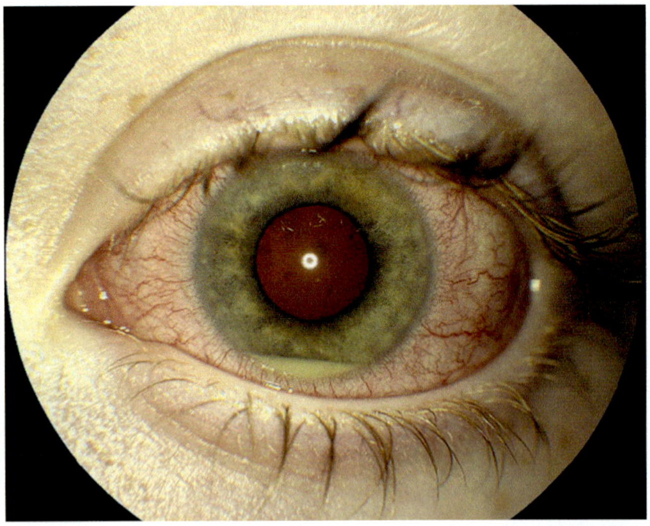

Fig. 9.15 A slit lamp colour image showing the anterior chamber of the left eye with pseudo-hypopyon during a hyperacute attack in a 13-year-old. This resolved completely with 3 days of systemic steroids

Table 9.10 Diagnostic criteria for IRVAN syndrome (Kincaid and Schatz 1983)

Major criteria	Minor criteria
Retinal vasculitis	Peripheral capillary non-perfusion
Neuroretinitis	Retinal neovascularisation
Aneurysmal dilations of the optic nerve head and retinal arterioles at or near their major branching sites	Macular exudation

neovascular glaucoma (Chang et al. 1995; Kincaid and Schatz 1983; Samuel et al. 2007; Rodríguez et al. 2019).

A staging classification was proposed in 2007 by Samuel et al. (See Table 9.11).

Patients without retinal neovascularisation and no visual loss can be considered for close observation (Chang et al. 1995; Basha et al. 2014) (See Fig. 9.17). However, pan-retinal photocoagulation (PRP) is standard treatment if there

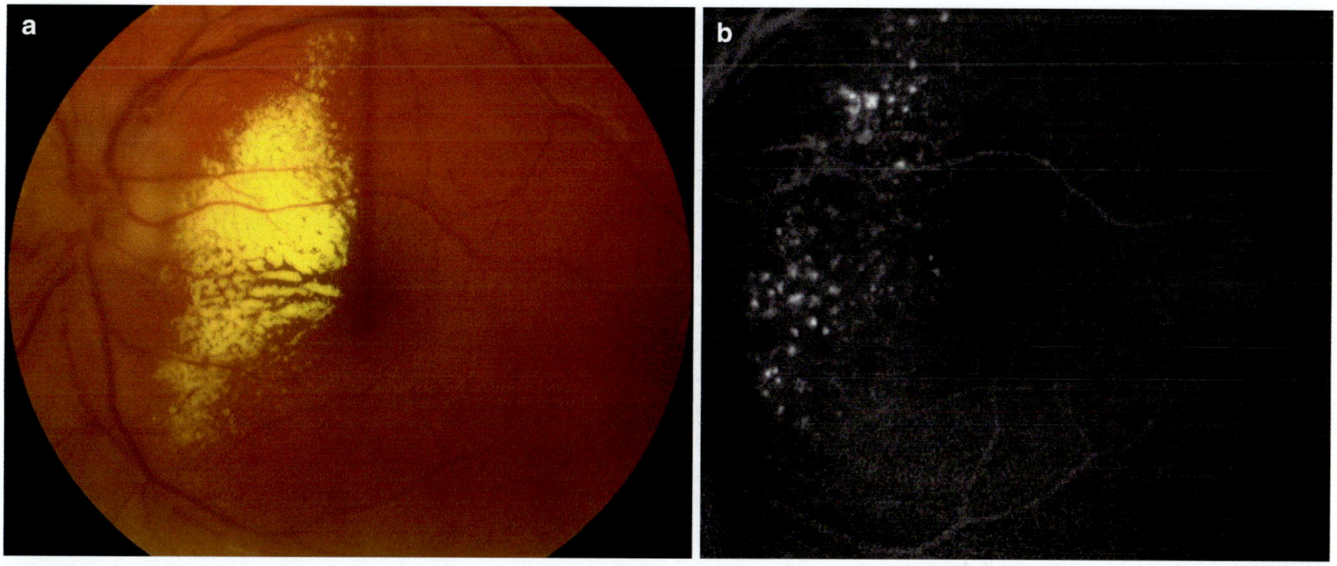

Fig. 9.16 (**a**) Shows a colour fundus photo of the left eye showing lipid depositions in the macula extending to the fovea, from a 10-year-old with normal vision. (**b**) Shows the corresponding FFA showing microaneurysms

Table 9.11 Staging classification for IRVAN syndrome developed by Samuel et al. (2007)

Stage	Ocular findings
1	Macroaneurysms, exudation, neuroretinitis, retinal vasculitis
2	Capillary nonperfusion with angiographic evidence
3	Posterior segment neovascularisation of disc or elsewhere and/or vitreous haemorrhage
4	Anterior segment neovascularisation
5	Neovascular glaucoma

is evidence of neovascularisation of the disc, neovascularisation elsewhere, or iris neovascularisation. PRP may also stop progression of the disease and can reduce the risk of further visual loss (Samuel et al. 2007). Unfortunately, due to the rarity of IRVAN, few high-quality studies have been done to assess the efficacy of any other treatments. Pars plana vitrectomy has been considered in eyes with vitreous haemorrhage and tractional retinal detachment, however, the case size is too small to draw any concrete conclusions (Samuel et al. 2007). A 0.7 mg dexamethasone intravitreal implant has been reported as a potential treatment (Empeslidis et al. 2013), as well as intravitreal ranibizumab (Karagiannis et al. 2010), and systemic infliximab (Cheema et al. 2011). However, these treatments have only been successful in small case series or case reports. Systemic corticosteroid use is controversial as oral steroids have not been shown to reduce the vasculitis or halt the progression of neovascularisation (Chang et al. 1995; Basha et al. 2014; Jones et al. 2000; Jyotirmay et al. 2010).

Ampiginous Choroiditis

Ampiginous choroiditis (AC) is a rare clinical entity first described by Jones et al. (2000), who termed it relentless placoid chorioretinitis, some ophthalmologists also consider ampiginous choroiditis a variant of serpiginous choroiditis (Lim et al. 2005). The term "ampiginous" was first coined by Nussenblatt and Whitcup (2010) by combining the acronym for acute posterior multifocal placoid pigment epitheliopathy (APMPPE) and the entity serpiginous choroiditis. AC has been described as resembling both APMPPE and serpiginous choroiditis showing similar clinical, indocyanine green angiography, and fluorescein findings (Jyotirmay et al. 2010). In the original case series, patients presented with a variety of symptoms with some patients having hyperaemia, some reporting decreased vision, and some reporting photopsias (Jones et al. 2000).

The etiology of AC is currently not clear due to its rarity and long disease course, tuberculosis has been put forward as a potential cause in endemic areas like India as this has been shown in serpiginous choroiditis (Cunningham et al. 2014; Mohan et al. 2014).

AC has plaque-like creamy white lesions at the level of the retinal pigment epithelium (RPE) not unlike the lesions found in APMPPE. Compared to APMPPE, AC has a higher number of lesions (>50), smaller placoid lesions (1/2 disc area), and lesions scattered around the posterior pole to the periphery and mid-periphery of the retina (Fig. 9.18). The lesions in AC are a mix of active and cicatricial lesions similar to serpiginous choroiditis. AC also shows a prolonged course with multiple flare ups; new lesions have been shown to appear up to 24 months after initial examination (Jones et al. 2000; Jyotirmay et al. 2010; Mirza and Jampol 2012).

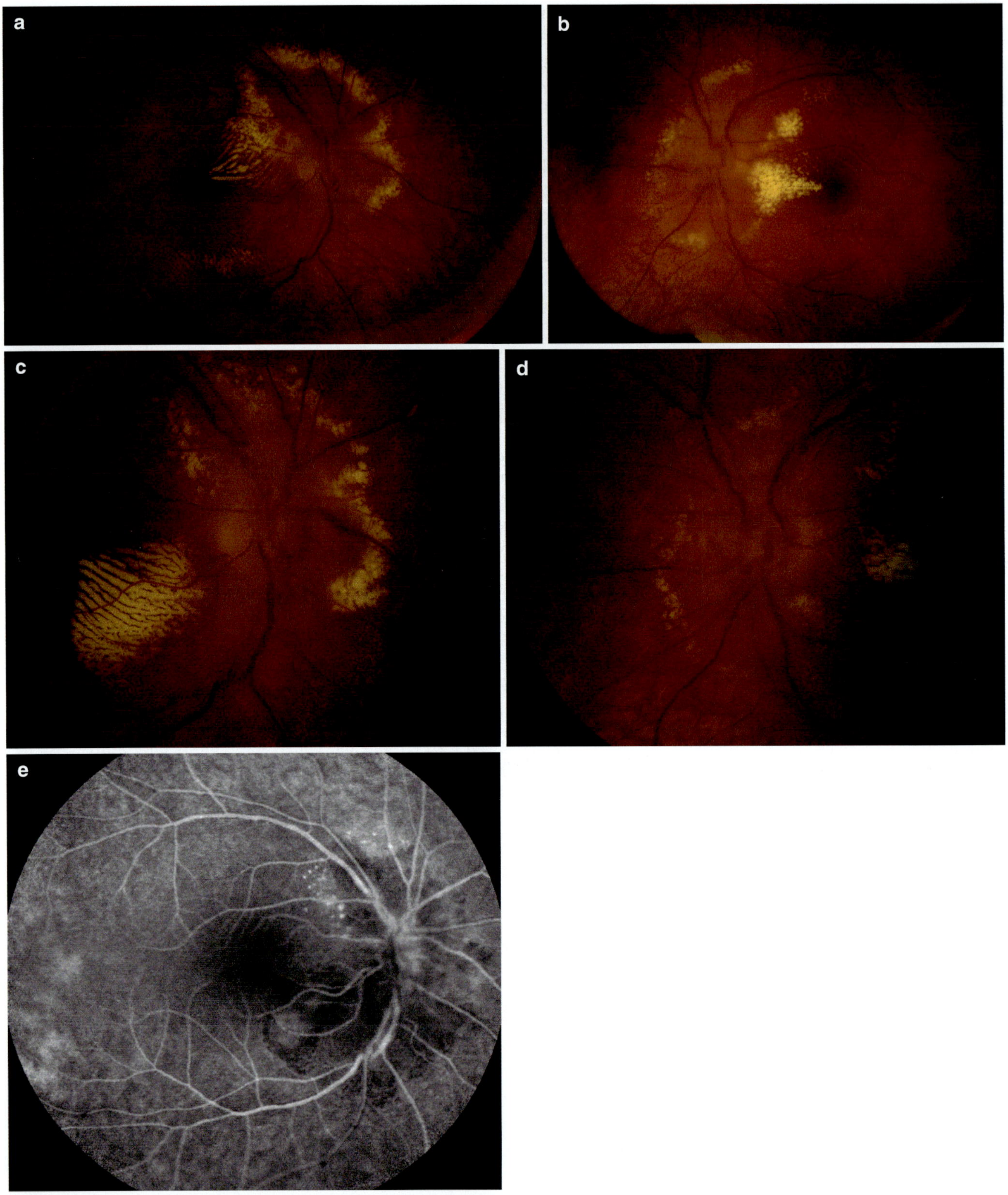

Fig. 9.17 (**a**) and (**b**) Colour fundus image of the right and left eye 1 year after initial presentation, vision remains normal at 6/6. (**c**) and (**d**) Colour fundus image of the right and left eye 2 years after initial presentation, the child remains asymptomatic with normal vision. (**e**) FFA of the right eye 3 years after initial presentation

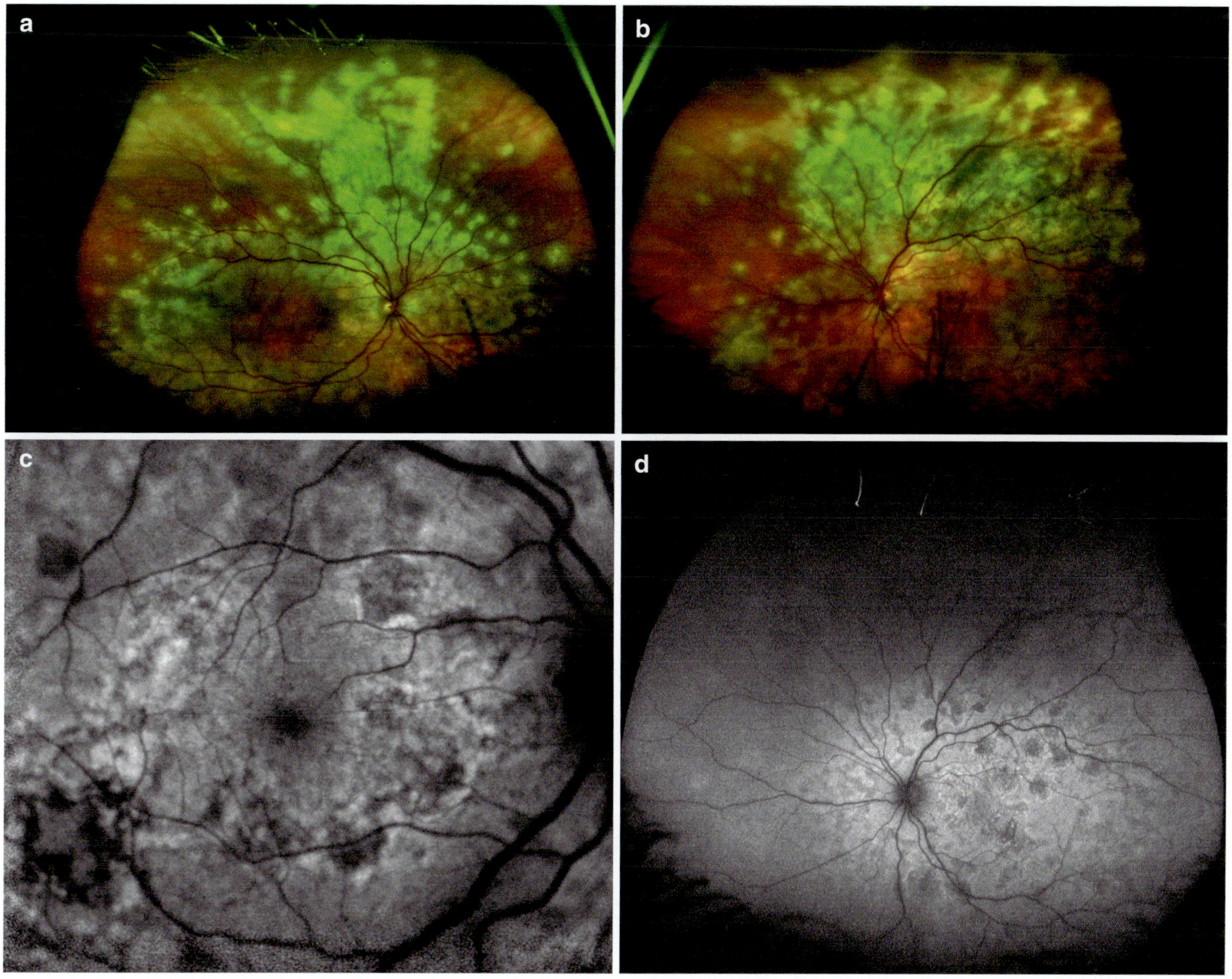

Fig. 9.18 (**a**) and (**b**) Optos fundus image of the right and left eye from a 14-year-old presenting with progressive sight loss to perception of light. All systemic work up for vasculitis and infective causes were negative including TB and HIV. (**c**) FFA of the right eye at onset. (**d**) Red free fundus image of the left eye at onset

The lesions develop at the level of the RPE and choriocapillaris with pigmentary disturbances remaining in AC compared to APMPPE where they resolve (Nazari Khanamiri and Rao 2013) (Fig. 9.19). Serpiginous choroiditis and APMPPE are extremely rare in children with very few cases having ever been reported.

A diagnostic criteria was made by Jyotirmay et al. in 2010 (Jyotirmay et al. 2010) (See Table 9.12).

Treatment for AC consists mainly of steroids and immunosuppressive therapy. Prognosis can depend on the location of the lesions, with a worse prognosis associated with lesions on the macula. Timely application of treatment is key to resolution of lesions in AC and recovery of vision (Jones et al. 2000; Jyotirmay et al. 2010).

Masquerade Syndromes

Neoplastic Masquerade Syndrome

Childhood neoplastic masquerade syndromes can emulate inflammatory conditions. Careful history, examination, investigations, and histopathologic evaluation of tissue specimens are required to make the correct diagnosis.

Retinoblastoma

Retinoblastoma is the most common ocular tumour in children under 5 years old, with an incidence of 1 in 15,000–20,000 worldwide (Kivelä 2009). It commonly presents as leukocoria. Other ocular features include conjunctival injection, hyphema, pseudo-uveitis, pseudo-hypopyon, and vitreous haemorrhage. Retinoblastoma looks distinctively

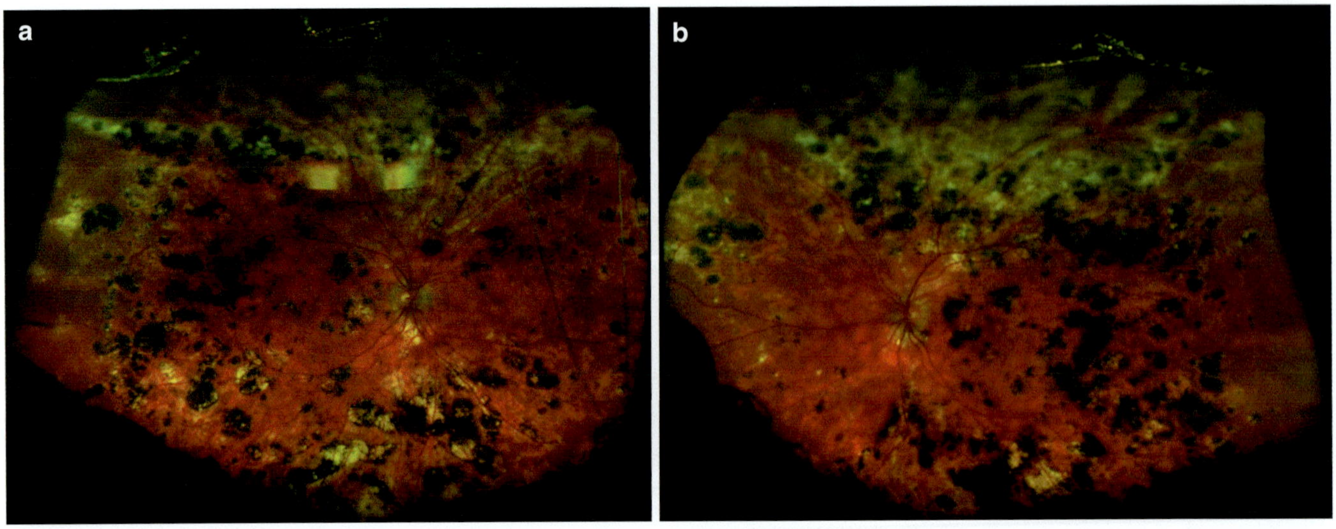

Fig. 9.19 (**a**) and (**b**) Optos fundus image of the right and left eye 3 years after presentation demonstrating hyperpigmented chorioretinal scars while vision is good at 6/6 in both eyes

Table 9.12 Diagnostic criteria for ampiginous choroiditis (Jyotirmay et al. 2010)

Diagnostic criteria
Yellowish-white placoid lesions with geographic borders occurring in the periphery and mid-periphery of the retina. Posterior pole may be involved later but rarely initially.
½ disc area lesions
Recurrent lesions
Fundus fluorescein angiography shows central hypofluorescence with hyperfluorescent margins.

different from retinitis, with fleshy raised retinal lesions affecting one or both eyes. It progresses rapidly and should not be confused with retinitis.

Acute Leukaemia

Acute leukaemia is the most common childhood cancer. Eye involvement can either be a result of direct leukaemic infiltration to the uvea, orbits, CNS, or secondary to haematological abnormalities (Bitirgen et al. 2016; Touhami et al. 2019).

Anterior segment infiltration is not common, reported in around 18% of cases, and it does not usually respond to steroid treatment (Wadhwa et al. 2007; Ramsay and Lightman 2001). Pseudo-hypopyon has been reported in children with acute lymphoblastic leukaemia (MacLean et al. 1996; Patel et al. 2003). Leukaemic retinopathy is the commonest presentation and reported in 70% of patients; this comprises of Roth's spots, retinal haemorrhages, perivascular sheathing, and cotton wool spots (Bitirgen et al. 2016; Patel et al. 2003). Choroidal infiltration can present as serous retinal detachment or drusen-like lesions; direct infiltration of the optic nerve can mimic papilloedema (Bitirgen et al. 2016; Sharma et al. 2004). Secondary opportunistic infections can create further challenges. Cerebral spinal fluid examination and neuroimaging are necessary to look for CNS infiltrates in children with ocular manifestations.

Diagnosis is confirmed by cytology of samples from the anterior chamber or vitreous. Ocular involvement may be the first and only sign in patients with relapse (MacLean et al. 1996). The management of childhood leukaemia requires close collaboration with paediatric oncologists in specialist centres.

Lymphoma

Lymphoma is the third most common form of childhood malignancy, accounting for 13% of newly diagnosed childhood cancers (Sandlund et al. 1996). 20% of patients with primary CNS lymphoma have ocular manifestations at diagnosis (Percy et al. 1999).

The most common ocular signs are vitritis associated with retinal/subretinal infiltrates, which give rise to the leopard skin appearance in the retina in an otherwise non-inflamed eye. Other less common presentations are pseudo-hypopyon and iris nodules that can mimic sarcoidosis.

Sudden loss of vision has been reported as a presenting symptom in young-onset non-Hodgkin lymphoma when the optic nerve is involved (Kourti et al. 2013). The diagnosis of intraocular lymphoma is based on clinical presentation and confirmed by pars plana vitrectomy with retinal or choroidal biopsy followed by cytology analysis.

Treatments include systemic and intrathecal chemotherapy. Irradiation of the globe and intravitreal chemotherapy such as methotrexate, rituximab, or daclizumab (Raja et al. 2013). Lymphoma, like other childhood onset cancers, remains an unpredictable and fatal condition despite advances in the management (Mărginean et al. 2018).

Paediatric oncologists must be involved in the management of these patients.

Non-neoplastic Masquerade Syndromes

Sympathetic Ophthalmia

Sympathetic ophthalmia (SO) is a rare bilateral non-necrotising granulomatous panuveitis, first described by Scottish ophthalmologist Sir William Mackenzie in 1830, then Fuchs in 1905 (Fuchs 1905; Mackenzie 1854). It has an incidence of 0.03/1,000,000 (Kilmartin et al. 2000). It is typically developed following penetrating injury or surgical procedure to one eye referred as the exciting eye, whereas the uninjured fellow eye is the sympathizing eye. The incidence has been reported to be higher in children at 0.24–1.4%, compared to 0.19% following penetrating eye injuries and 0.007% after ocular surgery, especially vitrectomy. The risk increases with consecutive eye surgeries, including non-penetrating ocular treatment such as cyclodestructive glaucoma procedures and ruthenium plaque brachytherapy in uveal melanoma (Edwards et al. 2014). The risk of developing SO is generally believed to reduce with early prophylactic enucleation of the blind excited eye with absolutely no vision potential, although the timing remains debatable.

The exact pathophysiology of SO is not confirmed but is generally agreed to be autoimmune, caused by a cell-mediated response to ocular antigens, such as S-antigen, inter-photoreceptor retinoid-binding protein, melanin associated antigens, and antigens derived from the RPE and choroid (Chu and Chan 2013).

Histologically, there is granulomatous infiltration of the uveal tract by lymphocytes, epithelioid cells, and multinucleated giant cells that may contain phagocytosed choroid and RPE; accumulated on the retinal phase of Bruch's membrane, clinically described as Dalen Fuch's nodules (Arevalo et al. 2012).

Development of SO has a genetic predisposition in those with HLA-A11, DRB1*04, DQA1*03, DQB1*04, D4, DQw3, DRw43, and patients with VKH disease (Shindo et al. 1997).

The onset of SO can be insidious or acute, it has been reported to start between 5 days and 66 years after the inciting event; with the majority presenting within 5 months of initial injury in children (Kumar et al. 2014). Patients with SO typically present with asymmetric bilateral panuveitis. Symptoms are usually more severe in the exciting eye ranging from minimal, to severe photophobia, floaters, and decreased vision.

Granulomatous uveitis features in SO include mutton fat keratic precipitates, posterior synechiae, glaucoma, vitritis, Dalen-Fuchs nodules (small yellowish pre-equatorial lesions), papillitis, and exudative retinal detachment (rarely retinal vasculitis) (Chu and Chan 2013). This can progress to cataracts, macular oedema, choroidal neovascularization, and optic atrophy. Extraocular findings including sensorineural deafness, alopecia, poliosis, and vitiligo are rare, but well-recognized features of SO.

Fluorescein fundus angiography (FFA) can be helpful, especially in milder cases, with early hypo- or hyperfluorescent RPE lesions, followed by late leakage and pooling of the dye in areas of exudative retinal detachment. The appearance of Dalen-Fuchs nodules simulates those seen in APMPPE. The optic nerve head may demonstrate leakage in the later stages of the angiogram. B-scan ultrasonography is useful in demonstrating the marked choroidal thickening seen in cases of SO (Chu and Chan 2013).

The diagnosis of SO is based on the history of eye trauma or surgery and clinical examination. There is no specific laboratory test to confirm. The clinical features can closely resemble VKH and other causes of granulomatous uveitis, such as sarcoidosis, while multifocal choroiditis can resemble APMPPE.

SO is a vision-threatening condition. Systemic steroids should be started early and used aggressively in order to avoid bilateral vision loss. Success has been reported in children with the use of biologic therapy such as adalimumab or infliximab, while a range of immunosuppressive agents has been reported to be effective such as azathioprine, cyclosporin, and interferon alpha (Kim et al. 2014; Gupta et al. 2011; Linda and Fardeau 2014). Therapeutic enucleation of the blind excited eye remains controversial after the process of SO has commenced, the beneficial outcome in saving the vision of the only functional sympathizing eye is difficult to prove, although this can be considered in refractory situations.

References

Abdelhakim A, Rasool N. Neuroretinitis: a review. Curr Opin Ophthalmol. 2018;29(6):514–9.

Abroug N, Khochtali S, Kahloun R, et al. Ocular manifestations of rickettsial disease. J Infect Dis Ther 2014;2(140):2332-0877.1000.

Achille M, Ilaria P, Teresa G, et al. Successful treatment with adalimumab for severe multifocal choroiditis and panuveitis in presumed (early-onset) ocular sarcoidosis. Int Ophthalmol. 2016;36(1):129–35.

Ahn SJ, Ryoo N-K, Woo SJ. Ocular toxocariasis: clinical features, diagnosis, treatment, and prevention. Asia Pacific allergy. 2014a;4(3):134–41. https://doi.org/10.5415/apallergy.2014.4.3.134.

Ahn SJ, Woo SJ, Jin Y, et al. Clinical features and course of ocular toxocariasis in adults. PLoS Negl Trop Dis. 2014b:8(6).

Allizond V, Costa C, Sidoti F, et al. Serological and molecular detection of Bartonella henselae in specimens from patients with suspected cat scratch disease in Italy: a comparative study. PLoS One. 2019;14(2):e0211945.

Almatary A, Bakir H. Human case of visceral larva migrans syndrome: pulmonary and hepatic involvement. Helminthologia. 2016;53(4):372–7.

Anand AR, Madhavan HN, Neelam V, et al. Use of polymerase chain reaction in the diagnosis of fungal endophthalmitis. Ophthalmology. 2001;108(2):326–30.

Andreoli CM, Foster CS. Vogt-Koyanagi-Harada disease. Int Ophthalmol Clin. 2006;46(2):111–22.

Ang M, Vasconcelos-Santos DV, Sharma K, et al. Diagnosis of ocular tuberculosis. Ocul Immunol Inflamm. 2018;26(2):208–16.

Arevalo JF, Garcia RA, Al-Dhibi HA, et al. Update on sympathetic ophthalmia. Middle East Afr J Ophthalmol. 2012;19(1):13.

Arnold SR, Ford-Jones EL. Congenital syphilis: a guide to diagnosis and management. Paediatr Child Health. 2000;5(8):463–9.

Aróstegui JI, Arnal C, Merino R, et al. NOD2 gene–associated pediatric granulomatous arthritis: clinical diversity, novel and recurrent mutations, and evidence of clinical improvement with interleukin-1 blockade in a Spanish cohort. Arthritis Rheum. 2007;56(11):3805–13.

Arun V, Noble AG, Group TS. Cataracts in congenital toxoplasmosis. J Am Assoc Pediatr Ophthalmol Strabismus. 2007;11(6):551–4.

Ash L. Ash and Orihel's Atlas of human parasitology. 5th ed. Chicago, IL: American Society for Clinical Pathology Press; 2007.

Azizlerli G, Akdağ Köse A, Sarıca R, et al. Prevalence of Behçet's disease in Istanbul, Turkey. Int J Dermatol. 2003;42(10):803–6.

Basha M, Brown GC, Palombaro G, et al. Management of IRVAN syndrome with observation. Ophthalmic Surg Lasers Imaging Retina. 2014;

Basu S, Kumar A, Kapoor K, et al. Neonatal endogenous endophthalmitis: a report of six cases. Pediatrics. 2013;131(4):e1292–e97.

Batts S, Demers DM. Spectrum and treatment of cat-scratch disease. Pediatr Infect Dis J. 2004;23(12):1161–2.

Behcet H. Uber rezidivierende, aphthose, durchein Virus verusachte Gaschwure am Mund, am Auge und an den Genitalien. Dermat Wochsch. 1937;105:1152–7.

Bhojwani R, Houtman AC, Stanga P, et al. Presumed early-onset sarcoidosis: a case of devastating ocular inflammation in an infant. J Pediatr Ophthalmol Strabismus. 2009;46(4):245–8.

Bitirgen G, Belviranli S, Caliskan U, et al. Ophthalmic manifestations in recently diagnosed childhood leukemia. Eur J Ophthalmol. 2016;26(1):88–91.

Blau EB. Familial granulomatous arthritis, iritis, and rash. J Pediatr. 1985;107(5):689–93.

Bosch-Driessen LH, Karimi S, Stilma JS, et al. Retinal detachment in ocular toxoplasmosis. Ophthalmology. 2000;107(1):36–40.

Bosch-Driessen LE, Berendschot TT, Ongkosuwito JV, et al. Ocular toxoplasmosis: clinical features and prognosis of 154 patients. Ophthalmology. 2002;109(5):869–78.

Boura P, Tselios K, Skendros P, et al. Adamantiades–Behçet disease (ABD) in northern Greece patients: experience from a single center. Hippokratia. 2007;11(4):210.

Braxton J, Davis DW, Emerson B, et al. Sexually transmitted disease surveillance 2017 2018. Atlanta: U.S. Department of Health and Human Services

Brunner J, Sergi C, Müller T, et al. Juvenile sarcoidosis presenting as Crohn's disease. Eur J Pediatr. 2006;165(6):398–401.

Carvalho R, Vazquez D, Silveira P, et al. Rickettsiosis: a rare challenge in ICU. Intensive Care Med. 2017;43(10):1514–5.

Caso F, Galozzi P, Costa L, et al. Autoinflammatory granulomatous diseases: from Blau syndrome and early-onset sarcoidosis to NOD2-mediated disease and Crohn's disease. RMD Open. 2015;1(1):e000097.

Chang TS, Aylward GW, Davis JL, et al. Idiopathic retinal vasculitis, aneurysms, and neuro-retinitis. Ophthalmology. 1995;102(7):1089–97. https://doi.org/10.1016/S0161-6420(95)30907-4.

Chang HK, Kim JU, Cheon KS, et al. HLA-B51 and its allelic types in association with Behçet's disease and recurrent aphthous stomatitis in Korea. Clin Exp Rheumatol. 2001;19(5):S24–31.

Cheema RA, Al-Askar E, Cheema HR. Infliximab therapy for idiopathic retinal vasculitis, aneurysm, and neuroretinitis syndrome. J Ocul Pharmacol Ther. 2011;27(4):407–10. https://doi.org/10.1089/jop.2010.0189.

Chen M, Sharifi E, Diaz V, et al. Combined systemic and intravitreal antiviral treatment in acute retinal necrosis. Invest Ophthalmol Vis Sci. 2016;57(12):4500.

Chi W, Yang P, Li B, et al. IL-23 promotes CD4+ T cells to produce IL-17 in Vogt-Koyanagi-Harada disease. J Allergy Clin Immunol. 2007;119(5):1218–24.

Chieffi PP, Santos SV, Queiroz ML, et al. Human toxocariasis: contribution by Brazilian researchers. Rev Inst Med Trop Sao Paulo. 2009;51(6):301–8.

Choukri F, Chakib A, Himmich H, et al. HLA-B∗ 51 and B∗ 15 alleles confer predisposition to Behçet's disease in Moroccan patients. Hum Immunol. 2001;62(2):180–5.

Chu XK, Chan C-C. Sympathetic ophthalmia: to the twenty-first century and beyond. J Ophthal Inflamm Infection. 2013;3(1):1–9.

Chung YM, Tsai ST, Liao F, et al. A genetic study of Behcet's disease in Taiwan Chinese. Tissue Antigens. 1987;30(2):68–72.

Cimaz R, Ansell B. Sarcoidosis in the pediatric age. Clin Exp Rheumatol. 2002;20(2):231–8.

Clarkson JG, Blumenkranz MS, Culbertson WW, et al. Retinal detachment following the acute retinal necrosis syndrome. Ophthalmology. 1984;91(12):1665–8.

Cunningham ET, Gupta A, Zierhut M. The creeping choroiditides – serpiginous and multifocal serpiginoid choroiditis. Ocul Immunol Inflamm. 2014;22(5):345–8. https://doi.org/10.3109/09273948.2014.962924.

Davatchi F, Shahram F, Chams H, et al. Pulse cyclophosphamide in ocular manifestations of Behcet's disease: a double blind controlled crossover study. 2004

Davatchi F, Shahram F, Chams-Davatchi C, et al. Behcet's disease: is there a gender influence on clinical manifestations? Int J Rheum Dis. 2012;15(3):306–14. https://doi.org/10.1111/j.1756-185X.2011.01696.x.

Davatchi F, Chams-Davatchi C, Shams H, et al. Adult Behcet's disease in Iran: analysis of 6075 patients. Int J Rheum Dis. 2016;19(1):95–103. https://doi.org/10.1111/1756-185X.12691.

de Melo Marques SH, Guerra MG, Almeida C, et al. Ocular manifestations of rickettsia in children: common but frequently overlooked. Case Rep. 2018;2018:bcr-2017-222809.

De-la-Torre A, Lopez-Castillo C, Gomez-Marin J. Incidence and clinical characteristics in a Colombian cohort of ocular toxoplasmosis. Eye. 2009;23(5):1090–3.

Desai SN, Pargewar SS, Agrawal N, et al. Hepatic visceral larva migrans with atypical manifestations: a report of three cases. Trop Gastroenterol. 2020;39(4):211–4.

Donahue SP, Greven CM, Zuravleff JJ, et al. Intraocular candidiasis in patients with candidemia: clinical implications derived from a prospective multicenter study. Ophthalmology. 1994;101(7):1302–9.

Drake WP, Newman LS. Mycobacterial antigens may be important in sarcoidosis pathogenesis. Curr Opin Pulm Med. 2006;12(5):359–63.

Du L, Kijlstra A, Yang P. Vogt-Koyanagi-Harada disease: novel insights into pathophysiology, diagnosis and treatment. Prog Retin Eye Res. 2016;52:84–111.

Dua S, Chalermskulrat W, Miller M, et al. Bilateral hematogenous Pseudomonas aeruginosa endophthalmitis after lung transplantation. Am J Transplant. 2006;6(1):219–24.

Eckert G, Melamed J, Menegaz B. Optic nerve changes in ocular toxoplasmosis. Eye. 2007;21(6):746–51.

Edwards JE Jr, Foos RY, Montgomerie JZ, et al. Ocular manifestations of Candida septicemia: review of seventy-six cases of hematogenous Candida endophthalmitis. Medicine. 1974;53(1):47–75.

Edwards J Jr. Candida species. Mandell, Douglas and Bennett's principles and practice of infectious diseases. 1995;4:2289–301.

Edwards TL, McKelvie P, Walland MJ. Sympathetic ophthalmia after diode laser cyclophotocoagulation: now an issue in informed consent. Can J Ophthalmol. 2014;49(4):e102–e04.

Eggimann P, Pittet D. Candida colonization index and subsequent infection in critically ill surgical patients: 20 years later. Intensive Care Med. 2014;40(10):1429–48.

Empeslidis T, Banerjee S, Vardarinos A, et al. Dexamethasone intravitreal implant for idiopathic retinal vasculitis, aneurysms, and neuroretinitis. Eur J Ophthalmol. 2013;23(5):757–60. https://doi.org/10.5301/ejo.5000301.

Engelhard SB, Bajwa A, Reddy AK. Causes of uveitis in children without juvenile idiopathic arthritis. Clin Ophthalmol (Auckland, NZ). 2015;9:1121.

Fauroux B, Clément A. Paediatric sarcoidosis. Paediatr Respir Rev. 2005;6(2):128–33.

Feigenbaum A. Description of Behçet's syndrome in the Hippocratic third book of endemic diseases. Br J Ophthalmol. 1956;40(6):355–7. https://doi.org/10.1136/bjo.40.6.355.

Fierro JL, Prasad PA, Fisher BT, et al. Ocular manifestations of candidemia in children. Pediatr Infect Dis J. 2013;32(1):84.

Figueira L, Fonseca S, Ladeira I, et al. Ocular tuberculosis: Position paper on diagnosis and treatment management. Revista Portuguesa de Pneumologia (English Edition). 2017;23(1):31–8.

Fink C, Cimaz R. Early onset sarcoidosis: not a benign disease. J Rheumatol. 1997;24(1):174–7.

Fisher M. Toxocara cati: an underestimated zoonotic agent. Trends Parasitol. 2003;19(4):167–70.

Flaxel CJ, Yeh S, Lauer AK. Combination systemic and intravitreal antiviral therapy in the management of acute retinal necrosis syndrome (an American Ophthalmological Society thesis). Trans Am Ophthalmol Soc. 2013;111:133.

Fuchs E. Über sympathisierende Entzündung (nebst Bemerkungen über seröse traumatische Iritis). Albrecht von Graefes Archiv für Ophthalmologie. 1905;61(2):365–456.

Ganatra JB, Chandler D, Santos C, et al. Viral causes of the acute retinal necrosis syndrome. Am J Ophthalmol. 2000;129(2):166–72.

Gandhi NR, Nunn P, Dheda K, et al. Multidrug-resistant and extensively drug-resistant tuberculosis: a threat to global control of tuberculosis. Lancet. 2010;375(9728):1830–43.

Gandhi TN, Slater LN, Welch DF, et al. Bartonella, including cat-scratch disease. Mandell, Douglas, and Bennett's principles and practice of infectious diseases. Elsevier; 2015. p. 2649–63.e4.

Ganesh SK, Bala A, Biswas J, et al. Pattern of pediatric uveitis seen at a tertiary referral center from India. Ocul Immunol Inflamm. 2016;24(4):402–9.

Garg S, Talwar D, Verma L. Metastatic endophthalmitis: a reappraisal. Ann Ophthalmol. 1991;23(2):74–8.

Garza-Leon M, Arellanes GL. Ocular toxoplasmosis: clinical characteristics in pediatric patients. Ocul Immunol Inflamm. 2012;20(2):130–8.

Gass JDM, Braunstein RA, Chenoweth RG. Acute syphilitic posterior placoid chorioretinitis. Ophthalmology. 1990;97(10):1288–97.

Gautam N, Singh R, Agarwal A, et al. Pattern of pediatric uveitis at a tertiary referral institute in North India. Ocul Immunol Inflamm. 2018;26(3):379–85.

Gazouli M, Ikonomopoulos J, Koundourakis A, et al. Characterization of Mycobacterium tuberculosis complex isolates from Greek patients with sarcoidosis by spoligotyping. J Clin Microbiol. 2005;43(9):4858–61.

Gedalia A, Khan TA, Shetty AK, et al. Childhood sarcoidosis: Louisiana experience. Clin Rheumatol. 2016;35(7):1879–84.

Gilbert R, Stanford M, Jackson H, et al. Incidence of acute symptomatic toxoplasma retinochoroiditis in south London according to country of birth. BMJ. 1995;310(6986):1037–40.

Greenwald MJ, Wohl LG, Sell CH. Metastatic bacterial endophthalmitis: a contemporary reappraisal. Surv Ophthalmol. 1986;31(2):81–101.

Griffin JR, Pettit TH, Fishman LS, et al. Blood-borne Candida endophthalmitis: a clinical and pathologic study of 21 cases. Arch Ophthalmol. 1973;89(6):450–6.

Grose C. Acute retinal necrosis caused by herpes simplex virus type 2 in children: reactivation of an undiagnosed latent neonatal herpes infection. Semin Pediatr Neurol. 2012;19(3):115–8.

Gül A. Pathogenesis of Behçet's disease: autoinflammatory features and beyond. Semin Immunopathol. 2015;37(4):413–8. https://doi.org/10.1007/s00281-015-0502-8.

Gupta V, Gupta A, Rao NA. Intraocular tuberculosis—an update. Surv Ophthalmol. 2007;52(6):561–87.

Gupta SR, Phan IT, Suhler EB. Successful treatment of refractory sympathetic ophthalmia in a child with infliximab. Arch Ophthalmol. 2011;129(2):250–2.

Habot-Wilner Z, Trivizki O, Goldstein M, et al. Cat-scratch disease: ocular manifestations and treatment outcome. Acta Ophthalmol. 2018;96(4):e524–e32.

Häfner R, Vogel P. Sarcoidosis of early onset. A challenge for the pediatric rheumatologist. Clin Exp Rheumatol. 1993;11(6):685–91.

Halperin JJ. Chronic Lyme disease: misconceptions and challenges for patient management. Infection Drug Resist. 2015;8:119.

Harada E. Acute diffuse choroiditis. Acta Soc Ophthalmol Jpn. 1926;30:356–78.

Harms A, Dehio C. Intruders below the radar: molecular pathogenesis of Bartonella spp. Clin Microbiol Rev. 2012;25(1):42–78.

Hawker JI, Bakhshi SS, Ali S, et al. Ecological analysis of ethnic differences in relation between tuberculosis and poverty. BMJ. 1999;319(7216):1031–4.

Hetherington S. Sarcoidosis in young children. Am J Dis Children. 1982;136(1):13–5.

Hillenkamp J, Nölle B, Bruns C, et al. Acute retinal necrosis: clinical features, early vitrectomy, and outcomes. Ophthalmology. 2009;116(10):1971–75.e2.

Hoffmann A, Milman N, Byg KE. Childhood sarcoidosis in Denmark 1979–1994: incidence, clinical features and laboratory results at presentation in 48 children. Acta Paediatr. 2004;93(1):30–6.

Holland GN. Standard diagnostic criteria for the acute retinal necrosis syndrome. Am J Ophthalmol. 1994;117(5):663–6.

Holland GN. Ocular toxoplasmosis: new directions for clinical investigation. Ocul Immunol Inflamm. 2000;8(1):1–7.

Holland GN. Ocular toxoplasmosis: a global reassessment: Part II: Disease manifestations and management. Am J Ophthalmol. 2004;137(1):1–17.

Hoover DL, Khan JA, Giangiacomo J. Pediatric ocular sarcoidosis. Surv Ophthalmol. 1986;30(4):215–28.

Hou S, Du L, Lei B, et al. Genome-wide association analysis of Vogt-Koyanagi-Harada syndrome identifies two new susceptibility loci at 1p31.2 and 10q21.3. Nat Genet. 2014;46(9):1007–11.

Houman MH, Neffati H, Braham A, et al. Behçet's disease in Tunisia Demographic, clinical and genetic aspects in 260 patients. Clin Exp Rheumatol. 2007;25(4):S58.

Hunninghake G, Costabel U, Ando M, et al. ATS/ERS/WASOG statement on sarcoidosis. American Thoracic Society/European Respiratory Society/World Association of Sarcoidosis and other Granulomatous Disorders. Sarcoidosis Vasculitis Diffuse Lung Dis. 1999;16(2):149.

Huppertz H-I, Münchmeier D, Lieb W. Ocular manifestations in children and adolescents with Lyme arthritis. Br J Ophthalmol. 1999;83(10):1149–52.

Ishida T, Sugamoto Y, Sugita S, et al. Prophylactic vitrectomy for acute retinal necrosis. Jpn J Ophthalmol. 2009;53(5):486–9.

Ishige I, Usui Y, Takemura T, et al. Quantitative PCR of mycobacterial and propionibacterial DNA in lymph nodes of Japanese patients with sarcoidosis. Lancet. 1999;354(9173):120–3.

Islam S, Numaga J, Fujino Y, et al. HLA class II genes in Vogt-Koyanagi-Harada disease. Invest Ophthalmol Vis Sci. 1994;35(11):3890–6.

Iwahashi C, Okuno K, Hashida N, et al. Incidence and clinical features of recurrent Vogt-Koyanagi-Harada disease in Japanese individuals. Jpn J Ophthalmol. 2015;59(3):157–63.

Iwahashi-Shima C, Azumi A, Ohguro N, et al. Acute retinal necrosis: factors associated with anatomic and visual outcomes. Jpn J Ophthalmol. 2013;57(1):98–103.

Jabs DA, Rosenbaum JT, Foster CS, et al. Guidelines for the use of immunosuppressive drugs in patients with ocular inflammatory disorders: recommendations of an expert panel. Am J Ophthalmol. 2000;130(4):492–513.

Jackson TL, Eykyn SJ, Graham EM, et al. Endogenous bacterial endophthalmitis: a 17-year prospective series and review of 267 reported cases. Surv Ophthalmol. 2003;48(4):403–23.

Jaeger EE, Carroll NM, Choudhury S, et al. Rapid detection and identification of candida, aspergillus, and fusarium species in ocular samples using nested PCR. J Clin Microbiol. 2000;38(8):2902–8.

Jennette JC, Falk RJ, Bacon PA, et al. 2012 Revised International Chapel Hill Consensus Conference Nomenclature of Vasculitides. Arthritis Rheum. 2013;65(1):1–11. https://doi.org/10.1002/art.37715.

Jones BE, Jampol LM, Yannuzzi LA, et al. Relentless placoid chorioretinitis: a new entity or an unusual variant of serpiginous chorioretinitis? Arch Ophthalmol. 2000;118(7):931–8.

Jyotirmay B, Jafferji SS, Sudharshan S, et al. Clinical profile, treatment, and visual outcome of ampiginous choroiditis. Ocul Immunol Inflamm. 2010;18(1):46–51.

Karagiannis D, Soumplis V, Georgalas I, et al. Ranibizumab for idiopathic retinal vasculitis, aneurysms, and neuroretinitis: favorable results. Eur J Ophthalmol. 2010;20(4):792–4. https://doi.org/10.1177/112067211002000425.

Karel I, Peleška M, Divišová G. Fluorescence angiography in retinal vasculitis in children's uveitis. Ophthalmologica. 1973;166(4):251–64. https://doi.org/10.1159/000306822.

Kawaguchi T, Hanada A, Horie S, et al. Evaluation of characteristic ocular signs and systemic investigations in ocular sarcoidosis patients. Jpn J Ophthalmol. 2007;51(2):121–6.

Kayes S, Oaks JA. Development of the granulomatous response in murine toxocariasis. Initial events. Am J Pathol. 1978;93(2):277.

Khairallah M, Ladjimi A, Chakroun M, et al. Posterior segment manifestations of Rickettsia conorii infection. Ophthalmology. 2004;111(3):529–34.

Khan A, Okhravi N, Lightman S. The eye in systemic sepsis. Clin Med. 2002;2(5):444.

Khan FA, Slain D, Khakoo RA. Candida endophthalmitis: focus on current and future antifungal treatment options. Pharmacotherapy J Hum Pharmacol Drug Therapy. 2007;27(12):1711–21.

Kilmartin DJ, Finch A, Acheson RW. Primary association of HLA-B51 with Behçet's disease in Ireland. Br J Ophthalmol. 1997;81(8):649–53.

Kilmartin DJ, Dick AD, Forrester JV. Prospective surveillance of sympathetic ophthalmia in the UK and Republic of Ireland. Br J Ophthalmol. 2000;84(3):259–63.

Kim B-S, Mehra S, Yawn B, et al. Increased risk of herpes zoster in children with asthma: a population-based case-control study. J Pediatr. 2013;163(3):816–21.

Kim J-B, Jeroudi A, Angeles-Han ST, et al. Adalimumab for pediatric sympathetic ophthalmia. JAMA Ophthalmol. 2014;132(8):1022–4.

Kincaid J, Schatz H. Bilateral retinal arteritis with multiple aneurysmal dilatations. Retina. 1983;3(3):171–8. https://doi.org/10.1097/00006982-198300330-00005.

Kirino Y, Bertsias G, Ishigatsubo Y, et al. Genome-wide association analysis identifies new susceptibility loci for Behcet's disease and epistasis between HLA-B*51 and ERAP1. Nat Genet. 2013a;45(2):202.

Kirino Y, Zhou Q, Ishigatsubo Y, et al. Targeted resequencing implicates the familial Mediterranean fever gene MEFV and the toll-like receptor 4 gene TLR4 in Behcet disease. Proc Natl Acad Sci. 2013b;110(20):8134–9.

Kivelä T. The epidemiological challenge of the most frequent eye cancer: retinoblastoma, an issue of birth and death. BMJ Publishing Group; 2009.

Koné-Paut I, Shahram F, Darce-Bello M, et al. Consensus classification criteria for paediatric Behçet's disease from a prospective observational cohort: PEDBD. Ann Rheum Dis. 2016;75(6):958. https://doi.org/10.1136/annrheumdis-2015-208491.

Kourti M, Mantadakis E, Anastasiou A, et al. Acute visual loss as the initial presentation in a child with systemic Burkitt lymphoma. Indian J Med Paediatr Oncol. 2013;34(2):99.

Koyanagi Y. Dysacousia, Alopecia und Poliosis bei schwere Uveitis nicht traumatischen Ursprungs. Klin Mblf Augenh. 1929;82:194–211.

Kumar K, Mathai A, Murthy SI, et al. Sympathetic ophthalmia in pediatric age group: clinical features and challenges in management in a tertiary center in southern India. Ocul Immunol Inflamm. 2014;22(5):367–72.

Kuo IC, Kapusta MA, Rao NA. Vitritis as the primary manifestation of ocular syphilis in patients with HIV infection. Am J Ophthalmol. 1998;125(3):306–11.

Kural-Seyahi E, Fresko I, Seyahi N, et al. The long-term mortality and morbidity of Behçet syndrome: a 2-decade outcome survey of 387 patients followed at a dedicated center. Medicine. 2003;82(1):60–76.

Kwon SI, Lee JP, Park SP, et al. Ocular toxocariasis in Korea. Jpn J Ophthalmol. 2011;55(2):143–7.

Latkany PA, Jabs DA, Smith JR, et al. Multifocal choroiditis in patients with familial juvenile systemic granulomatosis. Am J Ophthalmol. 2002;134(6):897–904.

Lim W-K, Buggage RR, Nussenblatt RB. Serpiginous choroiditis. Surv Ophthalmol. 2005;50(3):231–44.

Linda H, Fardeau C. Immunosuppressive treatment in Sympathetic ophthalmia: long-term visual outcome. Invest Ophthalmol Vis Sci. 2014;55(13):6299.

Lindsley CB, Petty RE. Overview and report on international registry of sarcoid arthritis in childhood. Curr Rheumatol Rep. 2000;2(4):343–8.

Liu Y, Zhang Q, Li J, et al. Clinical characteristics of pediatric patients with ocular toxocariasis in China. Ophthalmologica. 2016;235(2):97–105.

Mackenzie W. A practical treatise on the diseases of the eye. Longman, Brown, Green & Longmans; 1854.

MacLean H, Clarke MP, Strong NP, et al. Primary ocular relapse in acute lymphoblastic leukaemia. Eye. 1996;10(6):719–22.

Macpherson CN. The epidemiology and public health importance of toxocariasis: a zoonosis of global importance. Int J Parasitol. 2013;43(12-13):999–1008.

Madanat WY, Alawneh KM, Smadi MM, et al. The prevalence of Behçet's disease in the north of Jordan: a hospital-based epidemiological survey. Clin Exp Rheumatol. 2017;35(6):51–4.

Maitray A, Rishi E, Rishi P, et al. Endogenous endophthalmitis in children and adolescents: case series and literature review. Indian J Ophthalmol. 2019;67(6):795.

Manini MP, Marchioro AA, Colli CM, et al. Association between contamination of public squares and seropositivity for Toxocara spp. in children. Vet Parasitol. 2012;188(1-2):48–52.

Mărginean CO, Meliţ LE, Horvath E, et al. Non-Hodgkin lymphoma, diagnostic, and prognostic particularities in children–a series of case reports and a review of the literature (CARE compliant). Medicine. 2018;97(8)

Marshall GS, Stout GG, Jacobs RF, et al. Antibodies reactive to Rickettsia rickettsii among children living in the southeast and south central regions of the United States. Arch Pediatr Adolesc Med. 2003;157(5):443–8.

Martinez-Vaquez C, Fernandez-Ulloa J, Bordon J, et al. Candida albicans endophthalmitis in brown heroin addicts: response to early vitrectomy preceded and followed by antifungal therapy. Clin Infect Dis. 1998;27(5):1130–3.

Mathew RG, Goh BT, Westcott MC. British Ocular Syphilis Study (BOSS): 2-year national surveillance study of intraocular inflammation secondary to ocular syphilis. Invest Ophthalmol Vis Sci. 2014;55(8):5394–400.

Meghpara B, Sulkowski G, Kesen MR, et al. Long-term follow-up of acute retinal necrosis. Retina. 2010;30(5):795–800.

Mets MB, Chhabra MS. Eye manifestations of intrauterine infections and their impact on childhood blindness. Surv Ophthalmol. 2008;53(2):95–111.

Mikkilä HO, Seppälä IJ, Viljanen MK, et al. The expanding clinical spectrum of ocular lyme borreliosis. Ophthalmology. 2000;107(3):581–7.

Milman N, Selroos O. Pulmonary sarcoidosis in the Nordic countries 1950-1982. Epidemiol Clin Picture Sarcoidosis. 1990;7(1):50–7.

Mirza RG, Jampol LM. Relentless placoid chorioretinitis. Int Ophthalmol Clin. 2012;52:4.

Mochizuki M, Smith JR, Takase H, et al. Revised criteria of International Workshop on Ocular Sarcoidosis (IWOS) for the diagnosis of ocular sarcoidosis. Br J Ophthalmol. 2019;103(10):1418–22.

Mohan N, Balne PK, Panda KG, et al. Polymerase chain reaction evaluation of infectious multifocal serpiginoid choroiditis. Ocul Immunol Inflamm. 2014;22(5):384–90. https://doi.org/10.3109/09273948.2014.907433.

Moorthy RS, Inomata H, Rao NA. Vogt-koyanagi-harada syndrome. Surv Ophthalmol. 1995;39(4):265–92.

Mora P, Carta A. Ocular manifestations of Lyme borreliosis in Europe. Int J Med Sci. 2009;6(3):124.

Morelle G, Gueudry J, Uettwiller F, et al. Chronic and recurrent non-infectious paediatric-onset uveitis: a French cohort. RMD Open. 2019;5(2):e000933.

Moshfeghi AA, Charalel RA, Hernandez-Boussard T, et al. Declining incidence of neonatal endophthalmitis in the United States. Am J Ophthalmol. 2011;151(1):59–65.e1.

Muthiah MN, Michaelides M, Child CS, et al. Acute retinal necrosis: a national population-based study to assess the incidence, methods of diagnosis, treatment strategies and outcomes in the UK. Br J Ophthalmol. 2007;91(11):1452. https://doi.org/10.1136/bjo.2007.114884.

Mysterud A, Stigum VM, Jaarsma RI, et al. Genospecies of Borrelia burgdorferi sensu lato detected in 16 mammal species and questing ticks from northern Europe. Sci Rep. 2019;9(1):1–8.

Nagata K, Eishi Y, Uchida K, et al. Immunohistochemical detection of propionibacterium acnes in the retinal granulomas in patients with ocular sarcoidosis. Sci Rep. 2017;7(1):1–8.

Narendran N, Balasubramaniam B, Johnson E, et al. Five-year retrospective review of guideline-based management of fungal endophthalmitis. Acta Ophthalmol. 2008;86(5):525–32.

Nazari Khanamiri H, Rao NA. Serpiginous choroiditis and infectious multifocal serpiginoid choroiditis. Surv Ophthalmol. 2013;58(3):203–32. https://doi.org/10.1016/j.survophthal.2012.08.008.

Nelson KE, Williams CF. Early history of infectious disease: epidemiology and control of infectious diseases. Infect Dis Epidemiol Theory Pract. 2007:1–15.

Nelson CA, Saha S, Mead PS. Cat-scratch disease in the United States, 2005–2013. Emerg Infect Dis. 2016;22(10):1741.

Newman LS, Rose CS, Bresnitz EA, et al. A case control etiologic study of sarcoidosis: environmental and occupational risk factors. Am J Respir Crit Care Med. 2004;170(12):1324–30.

Noyola DE, Bohra L, Paysse EA, et al. Association of candidemia and retinopathy of prematurity in very low birthweight infants. Ophthalmology. 2002;109(1):80–4.

Nussenblatt RB, Belfort R. Ocular toxoplasmosis: an old disease revisited. JAMA. 1994;271(4):304–7.

Nussenblatt RB, Whitcup SM. Uveitis e-book: Fundamentals and clinical practice. Elsevier Health Sciences; 2010.

Ogura Y, Bonen DK, Inohara N, et al. A frameshift mutation in NOD2 associated with susceptibility to Crohn's disease. Nature. 2001;411(6837):603–6.

Ohno S, Ohguchi M, Hirose S, et al. Close association of HLA-Bw51 with Behçet's disease. Arch Ophthalmol. 1982;100(9):1455–8. https://doi.org/10.1001/archopht.1982.01030040433013.

Ohno S, Minakawa R, Matsuda H. Clinical studies of Vogt-Koyanagi-Harada's disease. Jpn J Ophthalmol. 1988;32(3):334–43.

Okada AA, Johnson RP, Liles WC, et al. Endogenous bacterial endophthalmitis: report of a ten-year retrospective study. Ophthalmology. 1994;101(5):832–8.

Okafuji I, Nishikomori R, Kanazawa N, et al. Role of the NOD2 genotype in the clinical phenotype of Blau syndrome and early-onset sarcoidosis. Arthritis Rheum. 2009;60(1):242–50.

Okhravi N, Adamson P, Mant R, et al. Polymerase chain reaction and restriction fragment length polymorphism mediated detection and speciation of Candida spp causing intraocular infection. Invest Ophthalmol Vis Sci. 1998;39(6):859–66.

Ombrello MJ, Kirino Y, de Bakker PIW, et al. Behçet disease-associated MHC class I residues implicate antigen binding and regulation of cell-mediated cytotoxicity. Proc Natl Acad Sci U S A. 2014;111(24):8867–72. https://doi.org/10.1073/pnas.1406575111.

Özdal PÇ, Ortaç S, Taskintuna I, et al. Long-term therapy with low dose cyclosporin A in ocular Behcet's disease. Doc Ophthalmol. 2002;105(3):301–12.

Paredes I, Ahmed M, Foster C. Immunomodulatory therapy for Vogt-Koyanagi-Harada patients as first-line therapy. Ocul Immunol Inflamm. 2006;14(2):87–90.

Parinaud H. Infective conjunctivitis of animal origin. Ann Ocul. 1889;101:252.

Parke DW II, Jones DB, Gentry LO. Endogenous endophthalmitis among patients with candidemia. Ophthalmology. 1982;89(7):789–96.

Patel SV, Herman DC, Anderson PM, et al. Iris and anterior chamber involvement in acute lymphoblastic leukemia. J Pediatr Hematol Oncol. 2003;25(8):653–6.

Pattishall EN, Kendig EL Jr. Sarcoidosis in children. Pediatr Pulmonol. 1996;22(3):195–203.

Percy C, Smith M, Linet M, et al. Lymphomas and reticuloendothelial neoplasms. Bethesda, MD: National Cancer Institute; 1999.

Perente I, Utine CA, Cakir H, et al. Management of ocular complications of Vogt-Koyanagi-Harada syndrome. Int Ophthalmol. 2009;29(1):33–7.

Peyron F, Garweg JG, Wallon M, et al. Long-term impact of treated congenital toxoplasmosis on quality of life and visual performance. Pediatr Infect Dis J. 2011;30(7):597–600.

Pikkel YY, Pikkel J. Acute retinal necrosis in childhood. Case Rep Ophthalmol. 2014;5(2):138–43.

Raja H, Snyder MR, Johnston PB, et al. Effect of intravitreal methotrexate and rituximab on interleukin-10 levels in aqueous humor of treated eyes with vitreoretinal lymphoma. PLoS One. 2013;8(6):e65627.

Rajendram R, Evans M, Rao NA. Vogt-Koyanagi-Harada disease. Int Ophthalmol Clin. 2005;45(2):115–34.

Ramsay A, Lightman S. Hypopyon uveitis. Surv Ophthalmol. 2001;46(1):1–18.

Rathi N. Current scenario of pediatric rickettsial diseases. Indian J Pediatr. 2016;83:1365–6.

Reiff A. Clinical Presentation, Management and Long Term Outcome of Pars Planitis (PP), Panuveitis (PU) and Vogt–Koyanagi–Harada disease (VKH) in Children and Adolescents. Arthritis Care Res. 2019;

Remmers EF, Cosan F, Kirino Y, et al. Genome-wide association study identifies variants in the MHC class I, IL10, and IL23R-IL12RB2 regions associated with Behcet's disease. Nat Genet. 2010;42(8):698–702.

Risseeuw S, de Boer JH, Ninette H, et al. Risk of rhegmatogenous retinal detachment in acute retinal necrosis with and without prophylactic intervention. Am J Ophthalmol. 2019;206:140–8.

Roach ES, Zimmerman CF, Troost BT, et al. Optic neuritis due to acquired toxoplasmosis. Pediatr Neurol. 1985;1(2):114–6.

Roberts F, Mets MB, Ferguson DJ, et al. Histopathological features of ocular toxoplasmosis in the fetus and infant. Arch Ophthalmol. 2001;119(1):51–8.

Rochlin I, Ninivaggi DV, Benach JL. Malaria and Lyme disease-the largest vector-borne US epidemics in the last 100 years: success and failure of public health. BMC Public Health. 2019;19(1):804.

Rodríguez Á, Carpio-Rosso W, Rodríguez FJ. Further observations on a bilateral IRVAN syndrome case. Int Ophthalmol. 2019;39(5):1179–86. https://doi.org/10.1007/s10792-018-0917-z.

Rolain J, Brouqui P, Koehler J, et al. Recommendations for treatment of human infections caused by Bartonella species. Antimicrob Agents Chemother. 2004;48(6):1921–33.

Rosé CD, Aróstegui JI, Martin TM, et al. NOD2-associated pediatric granulomatous arthritis, an expanding phenotype: study of an international registry and a national cohort in Spain. Arthritis Rheum. 2009;60(6):1797–803.

Rostami A, Riahi SM, Hofmann A, et al. Global prevalence of Toxocara infection in dogs. Adv Parasitol. 2020a;109:561.

Rostami A, Sepidarkish M, Ma G, et al. Global prevalence of Toxocara infection in cats. Adv Parasitol. 2020b;109:615.

Rothova A. Ocular involvement in toxoplasmosis. Br J Ophthalmol. 1993;77(6):371.

Roy R, Pal BP, Mathur G, et al. Acute retinal necrosis: clinical features, management and outcomes–a 10 year consecutive case series. Ocul Immunol Inflamm. 2014;22(3):170–4.

Rubinsky-Elefant G, Hirata C, Yamamoto J, et al. Human toxocariasis: diagnosis, worldwide seroprevalences and clinical expression of the systemic and ocular forms. Ann Trop Med Parasitol. 2010;104(1):3–23.

Rybicki BA, Iannuzzi MC. Epidemiology of sarcoidosis: recent advances and future prospects. Semin Respir Crit Care Med. 2007;28(1):22–35.

Rybicki BA, Iannuzzi MC, Frederick MM, et al. Familial aggregation of sarcoidosis: a case–control etiologic study of sarcoidosis (ACCESS). Am J Respir Crit Care Med. 2001;164(11):2085–91.

Saadoun D, Wechsler B, Terrada C, et al. Azathioprine in severe uveitis of Behçet's disease. Arthritis Care Res. 2010;62(12):1733–8.

Sadiq MA, Hassan M, Agarwal A, et al. Endogenous endophthalmitis: diagnosis, management, and prognosis. J Ophthal Inflamm Infection. 2015;5(1):1–11.

Sahu ES, Pal B, Sharma T, et al. Clinical profile, treatment, and visual outcome of ocular toxocara in a tertiary eye care centre. Ocul Immunol Inflamm. 2018;26(5):753–9.

Samuel MA, Equi RA, Chang TS, et al. Idiopathic retinitis, vasculitis, aneurysms, and neuroretinitis (IRVAN): new observations and a proposed staging system. Ophthalmology. 2007;114(8):1526–29.e1. https://doi.org/10.1016/j.ophtha.2006.11.014.

Sandlund JT, Downing JR, Crist WM. Non-Hodgkin's lymphoma in childhood. N Engl J Med. 1996;334(19):1238–48.

Sarens IL, Casteels I, Anton J, et al. Blau syndrome–associated uveitis: preliminary results from an international prospective interventional case series. Am J Ophthalmol. 2018;187:158–66.

Scherer WJ, Lee K. Implications of early systemic therapy on the incidence of endogenous fungal endophthalmitis. Ophthalmology. 1997;104(10):1593–8.

Schoenberger SD, Kim SJ, Thorne JE, et al. Diagnosis and treatment of acute retinal necrosis: a report by the American Academy of Ophthalmology. Ophthalmology. 2017;124(3):382–92.

Shah C, McKey J, Spirn M, et al. Ocular candidiasis: a review. Br J Ophthalmol. 2008;92(4):466–8.

Shakarchi FI. Ocular tuberculosis: current perspectives. Clin Ophthalmol (Auckland, NZ). 2015;9:2223.

Sharma T, Grewal J, Gupta S, et al. Ophthalmic manifestations of acute leukaemias: the ophthalmologist's role. Eye. 2004;18(7):663–72.

Shetty AK, Gedalia A. Childhood sarcoidosis: a rare but fascinating disorder. Pediatr Rheumatol. 2008;6(1):16.

Shields CL, Schoenberg E, Kocher K, et al. Lesions simulating retinoblastoma (pseudoretinoblastoma) in 604 cases: results based on age at presentation. Ophthalmology. 2013;120(2):311–6.

Shindo Y, Ohno S, Usui M, et al. Immunogenetic study of sympathetic ophthalmia. Tissue Antigens. 1997;49(2):111–5.

Shorbatli LA, Koranyi KI, Nahata MC. Effectiveness of antibiotic therapy in pediatric patients with cat scratch disease. Int J Clin Pharm. 2018;40(6):1458–61.

Silpa-archa S, Silpa-archa N, Preble JM, et al. Vogt–Koyanagi–Harada syndrome: perspectives for immunogenetics, multimodal imaging, and therapeutic options. Autoimmun Rev. 2016;15(8):809–19.

Silva RA, Berrocal AM, Moshfeghi DM, et al. Herpes simplex virus type 2 mediated acute retinal necrosis in a pediatric population: case series and review. Graefes Arch Clin Exp Ophthalmol. 2013;251(2):559–66.

Silveira C, Vallochi AL, da Silva UR, et al. Toxoplasma gondii in the peripheral blood of patients with acute and chronic toxoplasmosis. Br J Ophthalmol. 2011;95(3):396–400.

Simms I, Fenton KA, Ashton M, et al. The re-emergence of syphilis in the United Kingdom: the new epidemic phases. Sex Transm Dis. 2005;32(4):220–6.

Song Z, Marzilli L, Greenlee BM, et al. Mycobacterial catalase–peroxidase is a tissue antigen and target of the adaptive immune response in systemic sarcoidosis. J Exp Med. 2005;201(5):755–67.

Spagnolo P, du Bois RM. Genetics of sarcoidosis. Clin Dermatol. 2007;25(3):242–9.

Stanek G, Wormser GP, Gray J, et al. Lyme borreliosis. Lancet. 2012;379(9814):461–73.

Stanford M, Gilbert R. Treating ocular toxoplasmosis: current evidence. Mem Inst Oswaldo Cruz. 2009;104(2):312–5.

Stanford MR, Tan H-K, Gilbert R. Toxoplasmic retinochoroiditis presenting in childhood: clinical findings in a UK survey. Br J Ophthalmol. 2006;90(12):1464–7.

Steere AC, McHugh G, Damle N, et al. Prospective study of serologic tests for Lyme disease. Clin Infect Dis. 2008;47(2):188–95.

Sternberg P Jr, Han DP, Yeo JH, et al. Photocoagulation to prevent retinal detachment in acute retinal necrosis. Ophthalmology. 1988;95(10):1389–93.

Subauste CS, Ajzenberg D, Kijlstra A. Review of the series "Disease of the year 2011: toxoplasmosis" pathophysiology of toxoplasmosis. Ocul Immunol Inflamm. 2011;19(5):297–306.

Sykes RA, Makiello P. An estimate of Lyme borreliosis incidence in Western Europe. J Public Health. 2017;39(1):74–81.

Tabbara KF, Chavis PS, Freeman WR. Vogt-Koyanagi-Harada syndrome in children compared to adults. Acta Ophthalmol Scand. 1998;76(6):723–6.

Takeuchi M, Mizuki N, Meguro A, et al. Dense genotyping of immune-related loci implicates host responses to microbial exposure in Behçet's disease susceptibility. Nat Genet. 2017;49(3):438.

Tomassone L, Portillo A, Nováková M, et al. Neglected aspects of tick-borne rickettsioses. Parasit Vectors. 2018;11(1):263.

Touhami S, Audo I, Terrada C, et al. Neoplasia and intraocular inflammation: from masquerade syndromes to immunotherapy-induced uveitis. Prog Retin Eye Res. 2019;72:100761.

Touitou I, Koné-Paut I. Autoinflammatory diseases. Best Pract Res Clin Rheumatol. 2008;22(5):811–29.

Tugal-Tutkun I, Onal S, Altan-Yaycioglu R, et al. Uveitis in Behçet disease: an analysis of 880 patients. Am J Ophthalmol. 2004;138(3):373–80. https://doi.org/10.1016/j.ajo.2004.03.022.

Tugal-Tutkun I, Mudun A, Urgancioglu M, et al. Efficacy of infliximab in the treatment of uveitis that is resistant to treatment with the combination of azathioprine, cyclosporine, and corticosteroids in Behçet's disease: an open-label trial. Arthritis Rheum. 2005;52(8):2478–84.

Umran RM, Shukur ZY. Rituximab for sight-threatening refractory pediatric Vogt–Koyanagi–Harada disease. Mod Rheumatol. 2018;28(1):197–9.

Urayama A. Unilateral acute uveitis with retinal periarteritis and detachment. Rinsho Ganka (Jpn J Clin Ophthalmol). 1971;25:607–19.

Valbuena G. Rickettsioses: pathogenesis, immunity, and vaccine development. Acta Med Costarric. 2013;55:48–59.

Vallet H, Seve P, Biard L, et al. Infliximab versus adalimumab in the treatment of refractory inflammatory uveitis: a multicenter study from the French Uveitis Network. Arthritis Rheumatol. 2016;68(6):1522–30.

Van Gelder RN, Willig JL, Holland GN, et al. Herpes simplex virus type 2 as a cause of acute retinal necrosis syndrome in young patients. Ophthalmology. 2001;108(5):869–76.

Vogt A. Fruhzeitiges Ergrauen der Zilien und Bemerking uber den sogennanten plotzlichen eintritt dieser Veranderung. Klin Mblf Augenh. 1906;44:228–42.

Wadhwa N, Vohra R, Shrey D, et al. Unilateral hypopyon in a child as a first and sole presentation in relapsing acute lymphoblastic leukemia. Indian J Ophthalmol. 2007;55(3):223.

Watanabe T, Miki D, Okada A, et al. Treatment results for acute retinal necrosis. Nippon Ganka Gakkai Zasshi. 2011;115(1):7–12.

Weinberg R. Ocular involvement in Lyme disease. Am Acad Ophtalmol. 2008;

Wilder HC. Nematode endophthalmitis. Nematode endophthalmitis. 1950;

Won KY, Kruszon-Moran D, Schantz PM, et al. National seroprevalence and risk factors for zoonotic Toxocara spp. infection. Am J Trop Med Hygiene. 2008;79(4):552–7.

Wong J-S, Chan T-K, Lee H-M, et al. Endogenous bacterial endophthalmitis: an east Asian experience and a reappraisal of a severe ocular affliction. Ophthalmology. 2000;107(8):1483–91.

Wong R, Pavesio CE, Laidlaw DAH, et al. Acute retinal necrosis: the effects of intravitreal foscarnet and virus type on outcome. Ophthalmology. 2010;117(3):556–60.

World Health Organization. Global tuberculosis report 2013. World Health Organization; 2013.

Wouters C, Rose C. Childhood sarcoidosis. Handbook of Systemic Autoimmune Diseases. Elsevier; 2016. p. 427–49.

Yamada R, Kozono M, Ohmori T, et al. Simultaneous determination of residual veterinary drugs in bovine, porcine, and chicken muscle using liquid chromatography coupled with electrospray ionization tandem mass spectrometry. Biosci Biotechnol Biochem. 2006;70(1):54–65.

Yang P, Ren Y, Li B, et al. Clinical characteristics of Vogt–Koyanagi–Harada syndrome in Chinese patients. Ophthalmology 2007;114(3):606-14. e3.

Yazici H, Pazarli H, Barnes CG, et al. A controlled trial of azathioprine in Behcet's syndrome. N Engl J Med. 1990;322(5):281–5.

Yeshurun I, Recillas-Gispert C, Navarro-Lopez P, et al. Extensive dynamics in location, shape, and size of aneurysms in a patient with idiopathic retinal vasculitis, aneurysms, and neuroretinitis (IRVAN) syndrome. Am J Ophthalmol. 2003;135(1):118–20. https://doi.org/10.1016/S0002-9394(02)01823-8.

Yoshikawa K, Kotake S, Kubota T, et al. Cloning and sequencing of BES-1 gene encoding the immunogenic antigen of Streptococcus sanguis KTH-1 isolated from the patients with Behçcet's disease. Zentralblatt für Bakteriologie. 1998;287(4):449–60.

Yoshikawa M, Nishiofuku M, Moriya K, et al. A familial case of visceral toxocariasis due to consumption of raw bovine liver. Parasitol Int. 2008;57(4):525–9.

Young C, Lehner T, Barnes C. CD4 and CD8 cell responses to herpes simplex virus in Behçet's disease. Clin Exp Immunol. 1988;73(1):6.

Zhang T, Guo D, Xu G, et al. Ocular toxocariasis: long-term follow-up and prognosis of patients following vitrectomy. Ocul Immunol Inflamm. 2020;28(3):517–23.

Zouboulis CC. Epidemiology of Adamantiades-Behçet's disease. Ann Med Interne. 1999;150(6):488–98.

Zumla A, Raviglione M, Hafner R, et al. Current concepts. N Engl J Med. 2013;368:745–55.

Congenital X-Linked Retinoschisis

10

Prethy Rao, Vaidehi S. Dedania, and Kimberly A. Drenser

Introduction

Congenital X-linked retinoschisis (CXLRS) is an inherited retinal degeneration characterized by splitting of the superficial layers of retina. Although classically the nerve fiber layer is commonly split, separation of the retina may primarily involve any portion of the inner retina.

CXLRS was first described in two males by Haas (1898). Since then, it has been recognized by a variety of names, including neuroretinal disease in males, congenital cystic detachment of the retina, juvenile macular degeneration and congenital vascular veils. Jager coined the term "retinoschisis" in 1953 (Jager 1953) and presently the terms X-linked retinoschisis and juvenile retinoschisis are synonymous with CXLRS.

CXLRS is one of the most common juvenile macular degenerations. Depending on the population studied, the estimated prevalence of CXLRS ranges from 1 in 5000 to 1 in 20,000 (George et al. 1995a). CXLRS is a progressive disorder and other than ocular disease, there are no systemic associations.

Prethy Rao and Vaidehi S. Dedania contributed equally with all other contributors.

P. Rao
Royal Oak, MI, USA

V. S. Dedania
Royal Oak, MI, USA

Department of Ophthalmology, New York University, New York, NY, USA

K. A. Drenser (✉)
Royal Oak, MI, USA

Oakland University William Beaumont School of Medicine, Rochester, MI, USA
e-mail: kdrenser@arcpc.net

Etiopathogenesis

CXLRS is an X-linked recessive disorder usually affecting males. Females are rarely affected, although with lyonization or in cases of consanguinity or Turner's syndrome, females may manifest the disorder. CXLRS has complete penetrance, although there is variable expressivity. The cause of CXLRS has been tied to mutations in the retinoschisin 1 (RS1) gene on the distal short arm of the X chromosome (Xp22.1-p22.3), which encodes for the protein retinoschisin. Over 200 disease-causing mutations have been reported.

Retinoschisin is a 224 amino acid, discoid domain, secretory protein involved in cell-cell adhesion, and is expressed in photoreceptors, as well as in other components of the inner and outer retina, including ganglion cells, amacrine cells and bipolar cells. Thus mutations leading to CXLRS may affect the adhesive properties of retinoschisin in these various cell types (Molday et al. 2012; Grayson et al. 2000). Various cell types have been implicated as the primary cell involved in CXLRS, and to-date no studies have definitively identified any single cell. Early reports attributed many of the changes seen in CXLRS to gene defects in Muller cells, although other studies also implicate other retinal cells, such as photoreceptors and/or bipolar cells, in the pathophysiology. Studies in animal models have supported a role for retinoschisin in retinal maintenance, as there is continued expression. Although the molecular role of retinoschisin within the retina has not been completely elucidated, its interaction with β2 laminin may play a part in the pathogenesis of CXLRS (Libby et al. 1999).

The predominant disease-causing mutations are missense mutations, although null mutations and deletions have been described. Missense mutations in RS1 cause disease via interference with retinoschisin secretion, retinoschisin octamerization and/or protein function (Wu et al. 2005; Wang et al. 2006). These are believed to cause intracellular retention of retinoschisin. No correlation has been found between type of mutation and disease severity or prognosis,

R. V. P. Chan (ed.), *Pediatric Retinal Diseases*, Retina Atlas, https://doi.org/10.1007/978-981-19-1364-8_10

although some reports suggest milder disease in patients with missense mutations.

The pathophysiology underlying the formation of the schisis cavities in CXLRS remains unknown, although various theories have been proposed. Joshi et al. (2006a) suggested that at the structural level, vitreous tractional forces in combination with the intrastructural defects in retinoschisin might lead to schisis cavity formation. Others have postulated that the interaction between retinoschisin and the intracellular Na+/K+ ATPase pumps leads to an alteration in ionic gradients and tissue balance, resulting in extracellular fluid accumulation within the schisis cavities (Molday et al. 2012). Additionally, wide-field fluorescein angiography (FA) has shown vascular leakage, a potential source of schisis fluid (Rao et al. 2016).

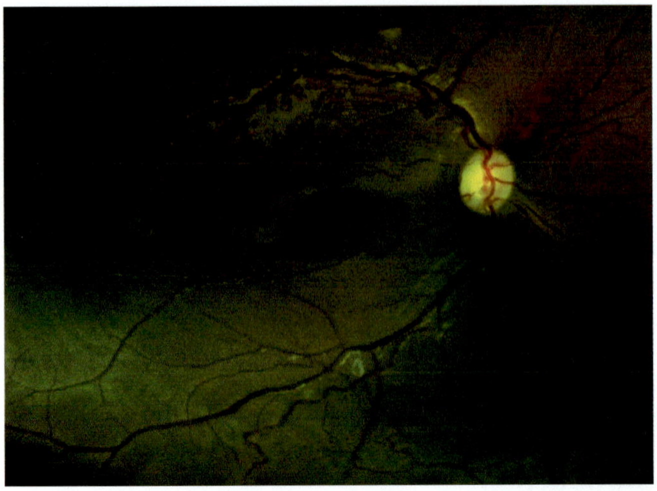

Fig. 10.1 Spoke-wheel pattern of foveal retinoschisis in a patient with congenital x-linked retinoschisis

Clinical Features

General Presentation

CXLRS occurs almost exclusively in males. Female carriers generally do not demonstrate fundus changes, although there are rare reports of heterozygotes with clinical signs (Gieser and Falls 1961; Wu et al. 1985). Affected male patients generally present in the first decade of life. While retinal findings have been described in infants at 3 months of age (Sieving et al. 1990), patients most commonly present at school age with impaired vision and strabismus. Visual impairment can vary drastically, with best-correct visual acuity ranging from 20/20 to 20/600, although typically vision is 20/60 to 20/120. Additionally, there is no consistency in visual impairment within a particular family or based on the type of mutation.

While there is a broad spectrum of clinical phenotypes in patients with CXLRS, a consistent feature of CXLRS in all affected males is "foveal schisis." Foveal schisis has a very distinct appearance of small cysts centered in the fovea and arranged in a stellate pattern or with radial striae, which on clinical examination can appear as a spoke-wheel pattern (Fig. 10.1). On initial examination, depending on age and disease status, foveal involvement may not be clinically apparent, although with imaging foveal schisis and/or retinal pigment epithelium (RPE) atrophy, resulting from previous schisis, may be visualized in the fovea. Only 50% of affected patients have peripheral retinoschisis, most commonly in the inferotemporal quadrant (George et al. 1995a).

Retinoschisis can be categorized as exudative and non-exudative. Eyes with exudative retinoschisis have lipid on examination (Fig. 10.2). One report described exudation in both the macula and periphery (Rao et al. 2016). It is unclear if the lipid in these patients is secondary to resolving hemorrhage, vascular incompetence, both or neither.

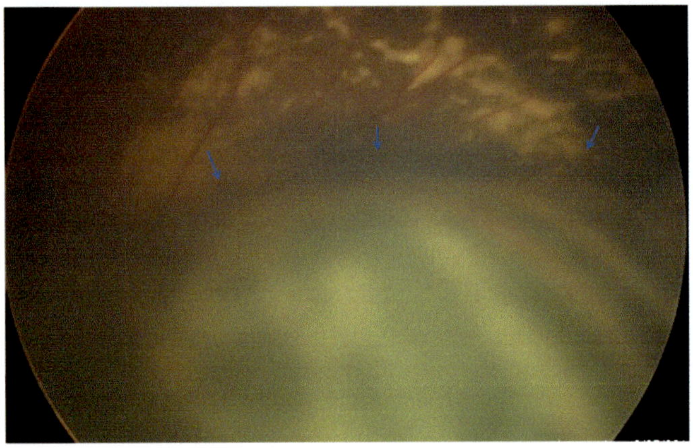

Fig. 10.2 Exudative congenital x-linked retinoschisis with peripheral bullous schisis overhanging the macula (arrows) and lipid

The inner retina may develop retinal holes or tears, or it may fragment over time, leaving membranous remnants (Fig. 10.3). Some use the term "vitreous veils" to describe these, although they are retinal or retinal and vitreal in nature and not only vitreous. In addition, the inner retina may or may not have retinal blood vessels. In some patients, the inner retinal vessels may cross into the vitreous, while in others, the retinal vessels may course in the outer leaf of the retina.

Patients may also develop optic disc and retinal neovascularization and may thus develop vitreous hemorrhage. The retina may also be dragged nasally, possibly secondary to the dehiscence of the nerve fiber layer temporally (Joshi et al. 2006a). Additionally, in some patients, the peripheral retina may also have a metallic sheen, RPE changes, intraretinal blood cysts or sheathed and occluded vessels (George et al. 1995a) (Fig. 10.4). A tapetal reflex associated with the Mizuo–Nakamura phenomenon has also been described.

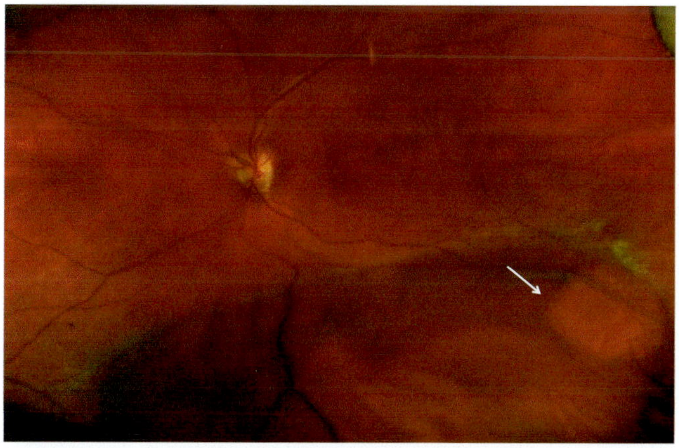

Fig. 10.3 Peripheral bullous retinoschisis with large inner wall hole (arrow) in a patient with congenital x-linked retinoschisis

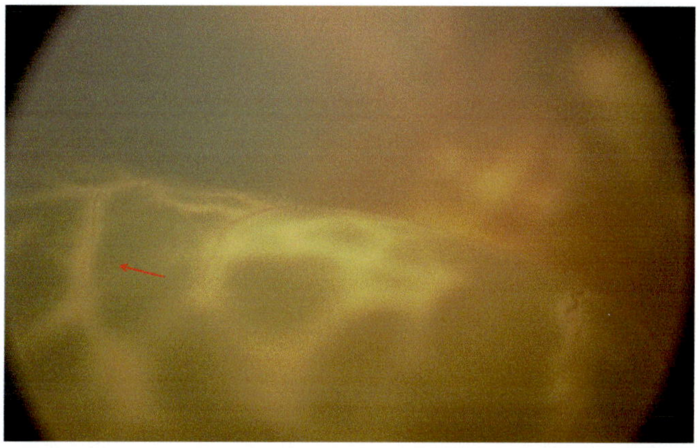

Fig. 10.4 Vascular sheathing in congenital x-linked retinoschisis

Natural History/Progression

The natural history of CXLRS varies considerably. Often, visual acuity deteriorates during the first and second decades of life and remains stable until the fifth and sixth decades. There are reports of bullous peripheral retinoschisis resolving spontaneously with apposition of the inner and outer retinal layers, occasionally leaving a pigment line.

The classic radiating striae evident in younger patients regresses with age, resulting in a blunted foveal reflex in older patients (Deutman 1971). RPE changes, in the macula and periphery and RPE atrophy, are also common in older patients, with macular atrophy as one of the most common causes for vision loss. The degenerative process in the macula can progress to loss of the photoreceptors and RPE, resulting in macular atrophy. Also with age, the intraretinal septae in the fovea can break down and the microcysts may coalesce, forming a large posterior schisis cavity, resulting in progressive loss of vision. Patients can develop vascular changes with age, such as sheathing of vessels and dendritiform patterns. Additionally, rarely, neovascular glaucoma can be seen.

Although the progression of vision loss in CXLRS is generally gradual, some patients may develop sudden vision loss secondary to retinal detachment and/or vitreous hemorrhage. Rhegmatogenous detachments develop secondary to outer retinal breaks in areas of peripheral schisis with concurrent inner retinal breaks or from full-thickness retinal breaks occurring during vitreous detachment. Others develop tractional retinal detachment from the retinoschisis cavity and/or posterior hyaloidal contraction. While pigment line is often associated with chronic retinal detachment, not all patients with CXLRS and chronic retinal detachment exhibit a pigment line. Similarly, chronic retinoschisis cavities without detachment can exhibit a pigmented demarcation line. Therefore, a pigment line cannot solely be used to include or exclude a chronic retinal detachment in these patients. Vitreous hemorrhage is a more common complication of CXLRS with an estimated incidence of 30–40% (George et al. 1995a). Hemorrhage can occur after bridging vessels rupture or secondary to neovascularization.

Diagnostic Imaging and Testing

Although the diagnosis of CXLRS is based on clinical examination, imaging, and other diagnostic testing has greatly improved our understanding of the disease. Patients with CXLRS demonstrate abnormalities on electroretinography (ERG), although none of them are unique to CXLRS, thus ERG is no longer the primary diagnostic tool utilized. On ERG in patients with CXLRS, there is a reduction in the dark-adapted b-wave amplitude, even in eyes with schisis confined to the fovea. Younger patients, in the early stages of disease, may have a normal a-wave, although with progressive involvement of the photoreceptors as patients age, there is reduction in the a-wave (Miyake et al. 1993). This combination of decreased b-wave amplitude and normal a-wave results in an electronegative ERG. Involvement of the inner and middle retina in CXLRS is also evident in the absence of the cone and rod oscillatory potentials and the scotopic threshold response on ERG (Peachey et al. 1987; Murayama et al. 1991). These changes indicate the possible role for other cells, such as amacrine cells, in disease pathogenesis. Patients may also have a reduced 30-Hz flicker response (Agarwal and Gass 2012). Obligate female carriers have not been consistently found have abnormalities on ERG. In young patients, there are often no changes on electro-oculography (EOG), although with progressive involvement of the RPE, the EOG is affected (Agarwal and Gass 2012).

On FA, there is no hyperfluorescence or leakage associated with the cystic-like spaces/retinal splitting in the fovea

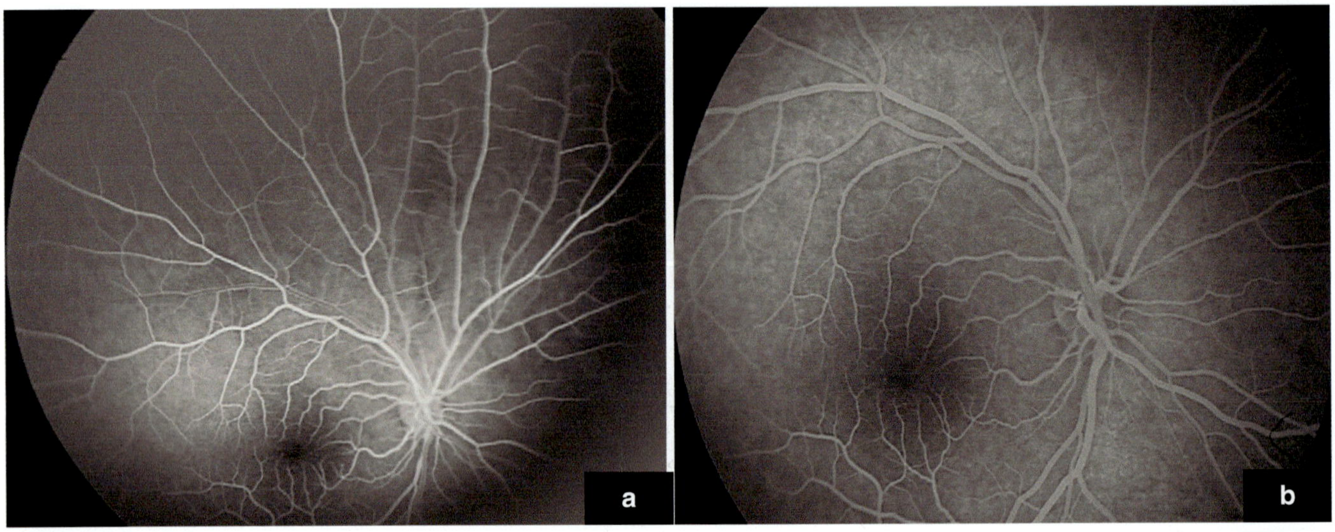

Fig. 10.5 (**a**) Early- and (**b**) late-phase fluorescein angiography of non-leaking foveal retinoschisis in a patient with congenital x-linked retinoschisis

(Fig. 10.5). This is in contrast to diabetic or classic cystoid macular edema where hyperfluorescence, secondary to leakage, is visualized on FA. Patients may occasionally have hyperfluorescence secondary to diffuse pigmentary changes or vascular leakage from retinal vessels within peripheral schisis. Additionally, some patients may demonstrate nonperfusion in both schitic and nonschitic areas.

With the advent of optical coherence tomography (OCT), the evaluation of patients with CXLRS has been enhanced drastically. OCT can demonstrate retinal splitting in patients with an apparently normal clinical exam. Additionally, it has shown that patients with CXLRS can have splitting in layers other than the nerve fiber layer. No studies have demonstrated a correlation between foveal appearance on OCT and visual acuity.

Genetic testing strategies include testing of just the RS1 gene or use of a multi-gene panel that includes RS1. If genetic testing in the proband yields a mutation in the RS1 gene, some defer genetic testing in others affected within the family, although the risk to siblings of the proband is dependent on the carrier state of the mother, and thus genetic testing is also recommended in the mother of the proband.

Classification

CXLRS has been classified into four phenotypes: type 1—foveal, type 2—foveo-lamellar, type 3—complex, and type 4—foveo-peripheral (Prenner et al. 2006) (Table 10.1). Type 1 CXLRS includes patients with only foveal schisis on clinical examination and optical coherence tomography (OCT). Macular lamellar schisis is recognized on OCT as macular schisis deeper than the nerve fiber layer outside the fovea in areas that appear normal on ophthalmoscopy. Foveo-lamellar CXLRS demonstrates foveal schisis on ophthalmoscopy and OCT and lamellar schisis on OCT without peripheral schisis on clinical examination (Fig. 10.6). Patients with type 3 CXLRS have involvement of all three retinal zones. These patients have foveal schisis on ophthalmoscopy and OCT, lamellar schisis on OCT and peripheral schisis on clinical examination. In foveo-peripheral (type 4), CXLRS ophthalmoscopy and OCT demonstrate foveal schisis and clinical examination shows peripheral schisis, but there is no lamellar schisis on OCT.

Table 10.1 Classification system for congenital X-linked retinoschisis

CXLRS type	Foveal cystic schisis (clinical examination)	Flat or lamellar macular schisis (OCT finding)	Peripheral schisis (clinical examination)
Type 1 foveal	+	−	−
Type 2 foveo-lamellar	+	+	−
Type 3 complex	+	+	+
Type 4 foveo-peripheral	+	−	+

CXLRS congenital X-lined retinoschisis, *OCT* optical coherence tomography

One study demonstrated type 3, complex, CXLRS as the predominant phenotype in 71% of patients (Prenner et al. 2006). The presence of retinoschisin in the inner and outer retina may account for the presence of lamellar schisis, deep

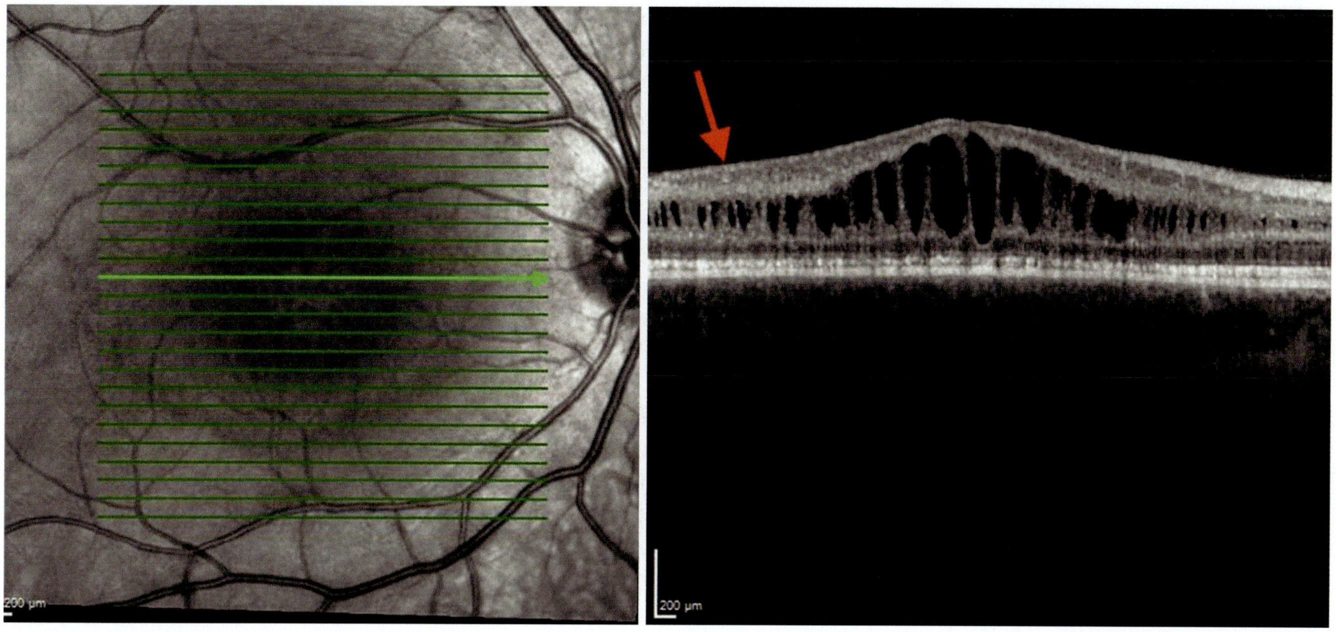

Fig. 10.6 Spectral domain-optical coherence tomography of the right eye in a patient with type 2—foveo-lamellar retinoschisis. The retinoschisis extends beyond the fovea (red arrow) with splitting of the retina in layers deep to the nerve fiber layer

to the nerve fiber layer. Currently, no studies have evaluated the prognostic significance of the various phenotypes of CXLRS.

Pathology

Histopathologically, retinal splitting occurs in the nerve fiber and ganglion cell layers. There are very few reports detailing the pathology of eyes with retinoschisis, especially in young eyes. In reports by Condon et al. (1986), patients had RPE degeneration only in areas with extensive photoreceptor cell degeneration. Additionally, the internal limiting membrane (ILM) overlying areas of retinoschisis was thinner than ILM overlying full-thickness retina.

At the molecular level, recent studies of schisis fluid have isolated cystatin C and tenascin-C, both involved in inflammation (Joshi et al. 2006a; Chiquet-Ehrisman and Chiquet 2003). Cystatin C is a protease inhibitor that is believed to protect tissues during pathologic conditions. On the other hand, tenascin-C may be adhesive and promigratory in one cell type but inhibitory in another. In contrast to patients with senile retinoschisis that have acid mucopolysaccharides in the schisis cavity, these have not been found in schisis cavities of patients with CXLRS. In one report, the histopathologic analysis revealed amorphous, eosinophilic PAS-positive, filamentous material, possibly originating from Muller cells within the schisis cavity (Kirsch et al. 1996). In another study, the intraretinal filaments isolated from schisis cavities were histologically distinct from filaments in the vitreous or material from typical cystoid degeneration or senile retinoschisis (Condon et al. 1986).

Management

The overall management of CXLRS is complex and depends on several factors, including disease severity, retinoschisis location and configuration, visual acuity and monocular status. Medical and surgical decisions can be divided into management of foveal retinoschisis, peripheral retinoschisis (extension into macula, overhanging macula), and/or CXLRS-related retinal detachments (combined rhegmatogenous schisis, combined tractional schisis).

Observation and Prophylaxis

Peripheral retinoschisis (with or without inner wall retinal breaks) that does not progress or extend into the macula is often observed given the low rates of progression. In our clinical experience, CXLRS-related retinal detachments (schisis RD) occur in less than 10% of patients. Hinds and colleagues report an 11% rate (2/18 eyes) of localized tractional schisis RD associated with peripheral retinoschisis, while the rates of rhegmatogenous schisis RDs range from 10 to 22% (Hinds et al. 2017; Ferrone et al. 1997).

Prophylactic treatment of peripheral retinoschisis is controversial, as spontaneous regression of retinoschisis cavities has been reported (George et al. 1995b). Prophylactic laser

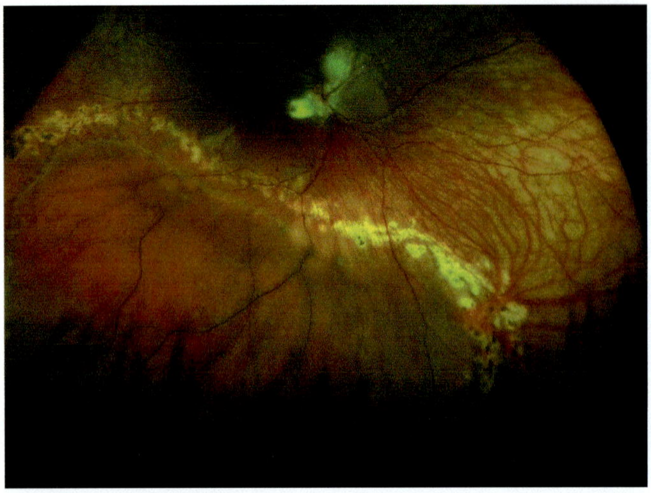

Fig. 10.7 Progressive peripheral bullous retinoschisis with barricade laser in a patient with congenital x-linked retinoschisis

barricade for stable peripheral retinoschisis is not recommended due to the high rates of iatrogenic retinal breaks and progression to rhegmatogenous schisis RDs (Brockhurst 1970). However, barricade laser photocoagulation—guided by optical coherence tomography, if available—with low power (<200 mW), long-duration burns (>300–400 ms) for progressive peripheral retinoschisis may be an alternative option in young patients that are unable to tolerate prolonged anesthesia or refuse surgery (Fig. 10.7). Prophylactic inner wall retinectomy or drainage has also been reported (Turut et al. 1989). However, in the absence of progression, the risk of a rhegmatogenous schisis RD or proliferative vitreoretinopathy (PVR) RD is a major concern (Turut et al. 1989; Sobrin et al. 2003). Therefore, prophylactic surgical intervention for stable peripheral retinoschisis is also not universally recommended.

Medical Management

Strabismus, amblyopia, and refractive errors (usually hyperopia) heavily contribute to the visual morbidity of CXLRS patients (Roesch et al. 1998; George et al. 1996). Therefore, the first and last steps are to maximize both strabismic management and refractive correction with a pediatric ophthalmologist. Currently, there are no clinical trials that support specific medical interventions for foveal CXLRS. Few case series have found success with topical carbonic anhydrase inhibitors (CAI) in the treatment of both foveal and peripheral retinoschisis (Verbakel et al. 2016; Sadaka and Sisk 2016; Ali and Seth 2013). Verbakel and colleagues most recently demonstrated a reduction in foveal zone thickness in five of nine patients (55.6%) with CXLRS after 6 months with oral CAI inhibitors (Verbakel et al. 2016). The exact mechanism is unknown, but several authors suggest target receptors in the RPE and neurosensory retina (Verbakel et al. 2016). However, the duration of treatment and safety profile requires further study. The use of ocriplasmin as primary treatment for macular schisis remains equivocal. One report suggests resolution after a single injection, however, the schisis recurred (Patel and Morse 2015).

Vitreoretinal Surgery Indications and General Principles

The decision for surgery in foveal or peripheral retinoschisis and CXLRS-associated retinal detachments is complex, multifactorial, and physician dependent. In the absence of a retinal detachment, monocular status, progressive vision loss, and retinoschisis configuration play key roles in surgical decision-making. A monocular patient with progressive vision loss in the better eye due to advancing peripheral retinoschisis will likely undergo a surgical intervention rather than observation. On the other hand, a young patient with either stable or slowly progressive vision changes in the weaker eye may warrant more extensive discussion with the family.

Posterior hyaloid separation is critical in CXLRS vitrectomy. The posterior hyaloid in pediatric patients is intimately adherent to the retina (Sebag 1991). Incomplete hyaloidal separation increases the risk of PVR and posterior hyaloidal contraction-related RDs (Joshi et al. 2006b; Drenser et al. 2016). Therefore, we first evaluate patients with rhegmatogenous schisis RDs for primary scleral buckling. Outer wall breaks are difficult to find, but are often located at the posterior edge of the schisis RD cavity.

If the rhegmatogenous schisis RD involves the macula, we will tend to proceed with a vitrectomy due to the difficulty in achieving proper support of posterior outer wall breaks with an encircling buckle. We advocate the use of ocriplasmin for posterior hyaloidal separation in progressive bullous peripheral retinoschisis, rhegmatogenous schisis and tractional schisis RDs (Wong and Capone 2013; Wu et al. 2007). Alternatively, two international units (IU, 0.1–0.2 mL) of plasmin enzyme isolated from 20 mL autologous blood 3 days prior to surgery are injected intravitreally 30 min prior to the vitrectomy (Wu et al. 2007). In the absence of ocriplasmin, indocyanine green (ICG), triamcinolone and/or perfluorocarbon (PFO) are also useful adjuncts for both vitreous dissection and identification of outer wall breaks. Ideally, we try to preserve the inner leaflet as much as possible in the hopes of using future gene therapy to reapproximating the inner and outer leaflets as noted below. However, if the posterior hyaloid cannot be separated from the inner schisis leaflet due to either an intimate adherence or thin inner leaflet, a limited inner wall retinectomy may be performed with or

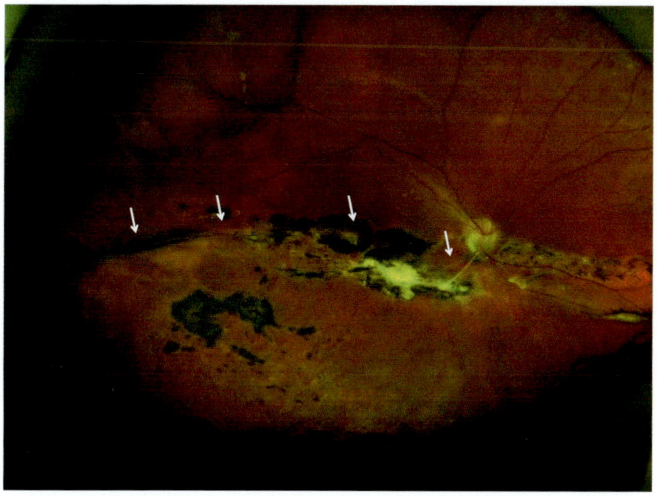

Fig. 10.8 Inner wall retinectomy (arrows) in a congenital x-linked retinoschisis-related rhegmatogenous retinal detachment

without light laser over the retinectomy and outer wall breaks (Trese and Ferrone 1995; Regillo et al. 1993) (Fig. 10.8). We typically perform an 80% silicone oil exchange for primary tamponade for several reasons: to achieve long-term stabilization of the schisis RD, to avoid postoperative positioning that is difficult to perform by children, to aid in dampening the potential for recurrent PVR, and to avoid elevated intraocular pressure and long-term corneal decompensation that can occur with silicone oil (Scott et al. 1999).

Foveal Retinoschisis

Foveal retinoschisis in the absence of a retinal detachment is often observed or treated medically first to avoid creating full-thickness retinal breaks associated with adherent posterior hyaloids intraoperatively. However, several reports suggest successful resolution of macular schisis with pars plana vitrectomy (PPV) (Byeon et al. 2007; Ikeda et al. 2008; Yu et al. 2012; Goel and Ghosh 2015). The exact mechanism is unknown, but a common theme among all reports suggests that foveal retinoschisis may have a structural component related to vitreoretinal traction from the internal limiting membrane (ILM) and/or posterior vitreous. Relief of these forces promotes resolution. Ikeda et al. demonstrated an 80% success rate (4/5 eyes) with collapse of macular retinoschisis after a pars plana vitrectomy, posterior vitreous detachment induction, ILM peeling and sulfur hexafluoride (SF6) tamponade (Ikeda et al. 2008). Iordanous confirmed this finding in a separate case report with ILM peeling (Iordanous and Sheidow 2013). Yu and colleagues published a prospective clinical series of 28 eyes that underwent observation ($n = 11$) or pars plana vitrectomy with careful limited ILM peeling around, but not involving, the foveal schisis ($n = 17$). In the surgical group, all eyes exhibited resolution of macular schisis, while nine eyes (82%) demonstrated progression in the nonsurgical group (Yu et al. 2012). Goel and Gosh reported the disappearance of foveal schisis after PPV and silicone oil tamponade with reappearance after oil removal (Goel and Ghosh 2015). Conversely, Gupta and colleagues reported an improvement in foveal cysts after scleral buckling for a CXLRS-related detachment (Gupta et al. 2015). Given the difficulty in removing all of the posterior hyaloid in pediatric patients and the risk of hyaloidal contraction, we recommend proceeding with caution when offering a PPV and including a thorough informed consent with the patient's family or legal guardian.

Peripheral Retinoschisis

Configuration and location of the peripheral retinoschisis are important for the surgical approach, decision for intervention, patient counseling and setting expectations for visual recovery. The presence of a demarcation line does not solely indicate the existence of a retinal detachment as it is present in patients with long-standing retinoschisis. In our experience, peripheral retinoschisis cavities with thin inner leaflets and inner retinal holes are more stable than cavities with smooth uninterrupted inner leaflets. Although the exact reason is unknown, free communication of fluid between the intraschisis cavity and vitreous with inner wall breaks may create a more stable vitreoretinal interface by equilibrating the push–pull forces between the schisis and vitreous cavities, respectively. Progressive bullous retinoschisis overhanging, but not involving, the macula may be amenable to vitrectomy. Surgical intervention for progressive peripheral retinoschisis involving the macula may have anatomic success, but visual success may be more unpredictable with a vitrectomy (Fig. 10.9). Our surgical technique for peripheral retinoschisis drainage begins with instillation of intravitreal ocriplasmin followed by a 23 or 25 gauge transconjunctival two or three-port vitrectomy approach. In the three-port technique, we use an anterior segment infusion cannula if the bullous schisis is retro-lenticular. After careful core and posterior vitreous hyaloidal separation, a small gauge cannula (42 gauge) is utilized to make a partial-thickness, inner wall drainage retinotomy in the schisis cavity to promote drainage under fluid–air exchange. An 80% silicone oil exchange is then performed for long-term tamponade. Garcia-Arumi and colleagues report a similar successful case (Garcia-Arumi et al. 2008). Armeda-Maresca and colleagues also published a variation of this technique by utilizing external drainage of bullous cavities abutting the lens in lieu of an internal partial-thickness drainage retinotomy (Armada-Maresca et al. 2011).

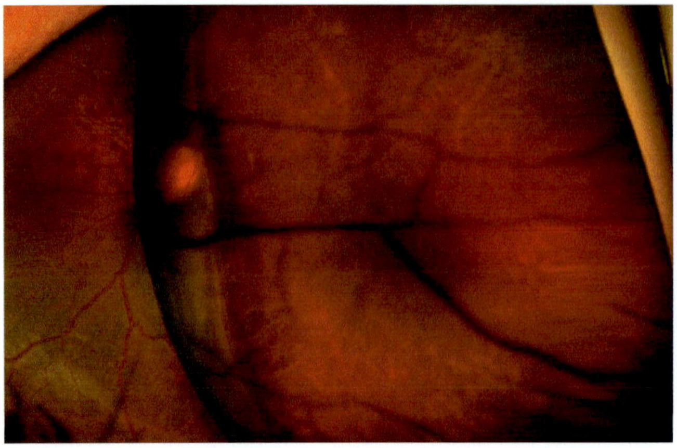

Fig. 10.9 Peripheral bullous retinoschisis overhanging and involving the macula in a patient with congenital x-linked retinoschisis

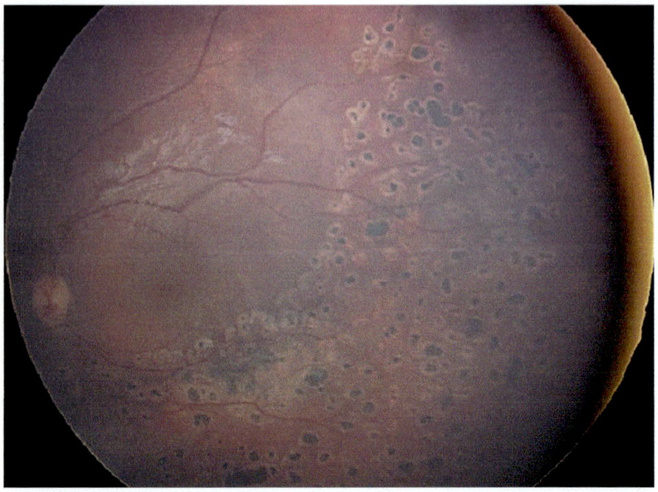

Fig. 10.10 Patient with congenital x-linked retinoschisis-related shallow rhegmatogenous retinal detachment that was treated with barricade laser

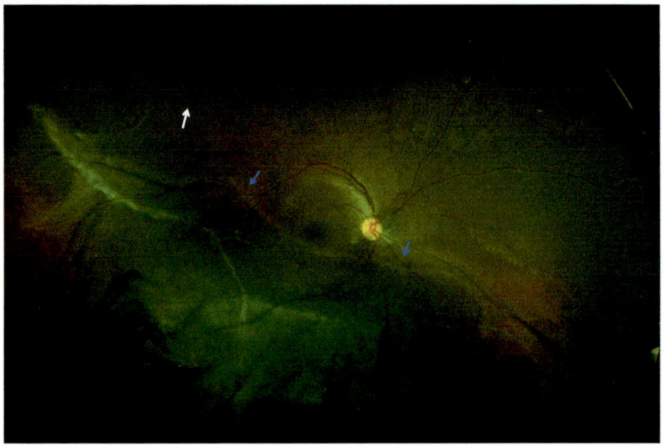

Fig. 10.11 Combined macula-involving rhegmatogenous schisis retinal detachment (blue arrows) in a patient with congenital x-linked retinoschisis with large inner wall holes (white arrow)

CXLRS-Related Rhegmatogenous and Tractional Retinal Detachments

Progressive macula-involving rhegmatogenous schisis RDs and tractional schisis RD may benefit from vitrectomy or scleral buckling, as discussed above. Additional indications include vitreous hemorrhage and exudative retinal detachments (Regillo et al. 1993; Rosenfeld et al. 1998; Schulman et al. 1985).

Although laser barricade is generally not recommended for peripheral retinoschisis, the role of laser photocoagulation for progressive rhegmatogenous schisis RDs is also controversial. We have found success in few cases of shallow combined rhegmatogenous schisis RDs with demarcation lines by careful green indirect laser photocoagulation starting at the posterior edge of the demarcation line and extending up to the ora serrata using long duration, low power burns (Fig. 10.10).

There are several reports that describe both scleral buckling and vitrectomy techniques for combined rhegmatogenous schisis RDs and tractional schisis RDs (Ferrone et al. 1997; Regillo et al. 1993; Rosenfeld et al. 1998). Surgically, we use a two or three-port technique after ocriplasmin with careful hyaloidal dissection for rhegmatogenous schisis RDs. We utilize triamcinolone, PFO, and ICG to assist in posterior hyaloid dissection as adjunctive agents, and PFO to help identify small peripheral outer wall breaks. If vitreous traction remains in rhegmatogenous schisis RDs, we proceed with an inner wall retinectomy and drain through the existing outer wall break with a large bore cannula followed by silicone oil tamponade (Fig. 10.11). A similar approach is utilized in PVR schisis RDs with careful peeling of the overlying proliferation in a posterior to anterior fashion using a combination of the Trese spatula and max grip forceps with or without PFO to both provide and control the degree of counter traction on the retina. In tractional schisis RDs in which a shallow macular RD is present but no outer wall break, vitrectomy is beneficial with careful hyaloidal dissection and internal drainage of the schisis cavity with a small gauge needle. In Type 2 or 3 CXLRS (unlike Type 4), we try to avoid inner wall retinectomies and dissect the anterior proliferation overlying the schisis cavity as the lamellar cavities are more difficult to separate from the deeper layers of the retina. However, it is not an absolute contraindication.

It is important to note that there is no single surgical approach or absolute guideline for CXLRS-related detachments due to the complexity of the anatomy and disease.

Future Gene Therapies

As retinoschisin is expressed in the retina during early development and maintained throughout life, gene replacement has become a target for therapeutic intervention. Gene replacement in CXLRS animal models has shown success in improving functional and structural deficits. Viral vector delivery of the RS1 gene in CXLRS mouse models shows promise as retinoschisin was successfully expressed in all retinal layers, and the b-wave amplitude was restored on ERG (Zeng et al. 2004; Min et al. 2005). Intravitreal injection of adeno-associated viral (AAV) vectors AAV8 and recombinant AAV2 (rAAV2) carrying functional RS1 into *Rs1*-deficient mouse models has demonstrated effectiveness. These are now currently being studies in human clinical trials. AAV8-mediated gene delivery in the *Rs1*-KO mice induced reorganization of the photoreceptor-depolarizing bipolar cell synapse and was found to restore function (Ou et al. 2015).

Currently, there are two gene therapy trials underway for the treatment of CXLRS. The National Eye Institute is conducting a phase I/II dose-escalation clinical trial for AAV8-scRS/IRBPhRS gene transfer in patients with CXLRS (NCT02317887). A biotechnology company, Applied Genetic Technologies Corporation (AGTC), is also performing a phase I/II dose-escalation clinical trial, for a rAAV2tYF-CB-hRS1 therapy (NCT02416622). Although both studies attempt to optimize dose, they are primarily designed to evaluate safety.

Other studies in animal models have used non-viral vectors for gene delivery. Apaolaza et al. (2016) used intravitreally administered solid lipid nanoparticles to induce retinoschisin expression in photoreceptors in *Rs1h*-deficient mice. They demonstrated structural improvement of the retina, with a decrease in cavities between the plexiform layers and bipolar cells, decreased photoreceptor loss and increased thickness of the outer nuclear layer and the retina (Apaolaza et al. 2016).

While these approaches show promise in animal models, application to humans may not be as successful as anticipated as there are significant differences in retinal pathogenesis and morphology. For example, the mouse models do not express any retinoschisin, while many patients with CXLRS have retinoschisin production, but abnormal protein structure and/or function. Such may interfere with wild-type protein generated from gene therapy. Another key difference in mice is that they lack a fovea, which is the target for visual improvement in humans. Although some animal studies have demonstrated improved ERG findings in treated patients, the functional impact of these treatments cannot be evaluated in these animal models. Finally, CXLRS is a rare disorder and recruitment for studies may be inadequate to accurately assess treatment efficacy and safety.

References

Agarwal A, Gass JDM. Chapter 5: Heredodystrophic disorders affecting the pigment epithelium and retina. In: Gass' atlas of macular diseases. London: Elsevier Saunders; 2012. p. 370–4. Print.

Ali S, Seth R. X-linked juvenile retinoschisis in females and response to carbonic anhydrase inhibitors: case report and review of the literature. Semin Ophthalmol. 2013;28(1):50–4.

Apaolaza PS, del Pozo-Rodreiguez A, Solinis MA, et al. Structural recovery of the retina in a retinoschisin-deficient mouse after gene replacement therapy by solid lipid nanoparticles. Biomaterials. 2016;90:40–9.

Armada-Maresca, Peralt-Calvo J, Pastora-Salvador N, Pulido JS, Fonseca-Sandomingo A. Combined external drainage and 25-gauge vitrectomy for severe X-linked congenital retinoschisis. Retina. 2011;31(6):1215–7.

Brockhurst R. Photocoagulation in congenital retinoschisis. Arch Ophthalmol. 1970;84(2):158–65.

Byeon SH, Lee SC, Koh HJ, Kim SS, Kwon OW. Surgical removal of the internal limiting membrane in progressive macular change in X-linked juvenile retinoschisis. Retin Cases Brief Rep. 2007;1(3):156–9.

Chiquet-Ehrisman R, Chiquet M. Tenascins: regulation and putative functions during pathological stress. J Pathol. 2003;200:488–99.

Condon GP, Brownstein S, Wang NS, Kearns JA, Ewing CC. Congenital hereditary (juvenile X-linked) retinoschisis. Histopathologic and ultrastructural findings in three eyes. Arch Ophthalmol. 1986;104:576–83.

Deutman AF. Sex-linked juvenile retinoschisis. In: Deutman AF, editor. The hereditary dystrophies of the posterior pole of the eye. Van Gorcum: Assen, the Netherlands; 1971. p. 48–98.

Drenser K, Girach A, Capone A Jr. A randomized, placebo-controlled study of intravitreal ocriplasmin in pediatric patients scheduled for vitrectomy. Retina. 2016;36(3):565–75.

Ferrone PJ, Trese MT, Lewis H. Vitreoretinal surgery for complications of congenital retinoschisis. Am J Ophthalmol. 1997;123(6):742–7.

Garcia-Arumi J, Corcostegui IA, Navarro R, Zapata MA, Berrocal MH. Vitreoretinal surgery without schisis cavity excision for the management of juvenile X-linked retinoschisis. Br J Ophthalmol. 2008;92(11):1558–60.

George ND, Yates JR, Moore AT. X-linked retinoschisis. Br J Ophthalmol. 1995a;79:697–702.

George NDL, Yates JRW, Bradshaw K, Moore AT. Infantile presentation of X-linked retinoschisis. Br J Ophthalmol. 1995b;79:653–7.

George ND, Yates JR, Moore AT. Clinical features in affected males with X-linked retinoschisis. Arch Ophthalmol. 1996;114:274–80.

Gieser EP, Falls HF. Hereditary retinoschisis. Am J Ophthalmol. 1961;51:1193–200.

Goel N, Ghosh B. Temporary resolution of foveal schisis following vitrectomy with silicon oil tamponade in X-linked retinoschisis with retinal detachment. Indian J Ophthalmol. 2015;63(11):867–8.

Grayson C, Reid SN, Ellis JA, et al. Retinoschisin, the X-linked retinoschisis protein, is a secreted photoreceptor protein, and is expressed and released by Weri-Rb1 cells. Hum Mol Genet. 2000;9:1873–9.

Gupta MP, Parlitsis G, Tsang S, Chan RV. Resolution of foveal schisis in X-linked retinoschisis in the setting of retinal detachment. J AAPOS. 2015;19(2):172–4.

Haas J. Ueber das Zusammenvorkommen von Veranderungen der Retina und Choroidea. Arch Augenheikd. 1898;37:343–8.

Hinds AM, Fahim A, Moore AT, Wong SC, Michaelides M. Bullous X linked retinoschisis: clinical features and prognosis. Br J Ophthalmol. 2017;

Ikeda F, Lida T, Kishi S. Resolution of retinoschisis after vitreous surgery in X-linked retinoschisis. Ophthalmology. 2008;115(4):718–22.

Iordanous Y, Sheidow TG. Vitrectomy for X-linked retinoschisis: a case report and literature review. Can J Ophthalmol. 2013;48(4):e71–4.

Jager GM. A hereditary retinal disease. Trans Ophthalmol Soc UK. 1953;73:617–9.

Joshi MM, Drenser K, Hartzer M, et al. Intraschisis cavity fluid composition in congenital X-linked retinoschisis. Retina. 2006a;26:S57–60.

Joshi MM, Ciaccia S, Trese MT, et al. Posterior hyaloid contracture in pediatric vitreoretinopathies. Retina. 2006b;26:S38–41.

Kirsch LS, Brownstein S, de Wolff-Rouendaal D. A histopathological, ultrastructural and immunohistochemical study of congenital hereditary retinoschisis. Can Ophthalmol. 1996;31:301–10.

Libby RT, Lavallee CR, Balkema GW, Brunken WJ, Hunter DD. Disruption of laminin beta2 chain production causes alterations in morphology and function in the CNS. J Neurosci. 1999;19:9399–411.

Min SH, Molday LL, Seeliger MW, et al. Prolonged recovery of retinal structure/function after gene therapy in an RS1h-deficient mouse model of X-linked juvenile retinoschisis. Mol Ther. 2005;12:644–51.

Miyake Y, Shiroyama N, Ota I, Horiguchi M. Focal macular electroretinogram in X-linked congenital retinoschisis. Invest Ophthalmol Vis Sci. 1993;34:512–5.

Molday RS, Kellner U, Bernhard HF, Weber BH. X-linked juvenile retinoschisis: clinical diagnosis, genetic analysis, and molecular mechanisms. Prog Retin Eye Res. 2012;31:195–212.

Murayama K, Kuo CY, Sieving PA. Abnormal threshold ERG response in X-linked juvenile retinoschisis: evidence for a proximal retinal origin of the STR. Clin Vis Sci. 1991;6:317–22.

Ou J, Vijayasarathy C, Ziccardi L, et al. Synaptic pathology and therapeutic repair in adult retinoschisis mouse by AAV-RS1 transfer. J Clin Invest. 2015;125:2891–903.

Patel A, Morse L. Ocriplasmin for foveal schisis in X-linked retinoschisis. Retin Cases Brief Rep. 2015;9(3):248–51.

Peachey NS, Fishman GA, Derlacki DJ, Brigell MG. Psychophysical and electroretinographic findings in X-linked juvenile retinoschisis. Arch Ophthalmol. 1987;105:513–6.

Prenner JL, Capone A Jr, Ciaccia S, et al. Congenital X-linked retinoschisis cslassification system. Retina. 2006;26:S61–4.

Rao P, Robinson J, Yonekawa Y, et al. Wide-field imaging of nonexudative and exudative congenital X-linked retinoschisis. Retina. 2016;36:1093–100.

Regillo CD, Tasman WS, Brown GC. Surgical management of complications associated with X-linked retinoschisis. Arch Ophthalmol. 1993;111(8):1080–6.

Roesch MT, Ewing CC, Gibson AE, et al. The natural history of X-linked retinoschisis. Can J Ophthalmol. 1998;33:149–58.

Rosenfeld PJ, Flynn HW Jr, McDonald HR, et al. Outcomes of vitreoretinal surgery in patients with X-linked retinoschisis. Ophthalmic Surg Lasers. 1998;29(3):190–7.

Sadaka A, Sisk RA. Dramatic regression of macular and peripheral retinoschisis with dorzolamide 2% in X-linked retinoschisis: a case report. J Med Case Rep. 2016;10(1):142.

Schulman J, Peyman GA, Jednock N, Larson B. Indications for vitrectomy in congenital retinoschisis. Br J Ophthalmol. 1985;69(7):482–6.

Scott IU, Flynn HW, Azen SP, et al. Silicone oil in the repair of pediatric complex retinal detachments: a prospective, observational, multicenter study. Ophthalmology. 1999;106(7):1399–407; discussion 1407–8.

Sebag J. Age-related differences in the human vitreoretinal interface. Arch Ophthalmol. 1991;109:966–71.

Sieving PA, Bingham EL, Roth MS, et al. Linkage relationship of X-linked juvenile retinoschisis with Xp22.1–p22.3 probes. Am J Hum Genet. 1990:616–21.

Sobrin L, Berrocal AM, Murray TG. Retinal detachment 7 years after prophylactic schisis cavity excision in juvenile X-linked retinoschisis. Ophthalmic Surg Lasers Imaging. 2003;34(5):401–2.

Trese MT, Ferrone PJ. The role of inner wall retinectomy in the management of juvenile retinoschisis. Graefes Arch Clin Exp Ophthalmol. 1995;233(11):706–8.

Turut P, Francois P, Castier P, Milazzo S. Analysis of results in the treatment of peripheral retinoschisis in sex-linked congenital retinoschisis. Graefes Arch Clin Exp Ophthalmol. 1989;227(4):328–31.

Verbakel SK, van de Ven JP, Le Blanc LM, Groenwoud JM, de Jong EK, Klevering BJ, Hoyng CB. Carbonic anhydrase inhibitors for the treatment of cystic macular lesions in children with x-linked juvenile retinoschisis. Invest Ophthalmol Vis Sci. 2016;57(13):5143–7.

Wang T, Zhou A, Waters CT, O'Connor E, Read RJ, Trump D. Molecular pathology of X linked retinoschisis: mutations interfere with retinoschisin secretion and oligomerisation. Br J Ophthalmol. 2006;90:81–6.

Wong SC, Capone A Jr. Microplasmin (ocriplasmin) in pediatric vitreoretinal surgery: update and review. Retina. 2013;33(2):339–48.

Wu G, Cotlier E, Braudie S. A carrier state of X-linked juvenile retinoschisis. Ophthalmic Paediatr Genet. 1985;5:13–7.

Wu WW, Wong JP, Kast J, Molday RS. RS1, a discoidin domain-containing retinal cell adhesion protein associated with X-linked retinoschisis, exists as a novel disulfide-linked octamer. J Biol Chem. 2005;280:10721–30.

Wu WC, Drenser KA, Capone A Jr, Williams GA, Trese MT. Plasmin enzyme-assisted vitreoretinal surgery in congenital X-linked retinoschisis: surgical techniques based on a new classification system. Retina. 2007;27(8):1079–85.

Yu H, Li T, Luo Y, et al. Long-term outcomes of vitrectomy for progressive X-linked retinoschisis. Am J Ophthalmol. 2012;154(2):394–402.

Zeng Y, Takada Y, Kjellstrom S, et al. RS-1 Gene delivery to an adult RS1h knockout mouse model restores ERG b-wave with reversal of the electronegative waveform of X-linked retinoschisis. Invest Ophthalmol Vis Sci. 2004;45(9):3279–85.

Hematologic Disorders: Leukemia, Hyperviscosity, Anemia

11

Tomas Moreno, Stephen J. Kim, and Ingrid U. Scott

Leukemia is the most common cancer in the pediatric population, accounting for nearly one out of three pediatric cancers. Most childhood leukemias are acute lymphocytic leukemia (ALL) and the remaining are acute myeloid leukemia (AML). In contrast, chronic leukemias are rare in childhood. Ocular findings are varied, but the retina is the most commonly involved tissue site in clinical studies. While direct retinal invasion by leukemic cells can occur, the majority of retinal findings are likely due to secondary hematologic changes. The term leukemic retinopathy often describes the manifestation of anemia and increased blood viscosity in patients with leukemia and are, therefore, topics included for review below.

Introduction

Hematologic disorders have a wide variety of presentations in the retina. More common hematologic disorders include leukemia, hyperviscosity syndrome, and anemia. Awareness of their associated retinal findings is important to facilitate timely diagnosis.

The prevalence of ocular manifestations in patients with leukemia can be as high as 90% and mostly effect the retina (Kincaid and Green 1983). These findings can result from direct invasion of neoplastic cells or result from secondary consequences of leukemia such as anemia, thrombocytopenia (Fig. 11.1), or hyperviscosity. Other hyperviscosity syndromes or conditions that result in anemia have similar retinal manifestations. In this chapter, we will describe leukemia and its retinal manifestations. We will also describe retinal findings associated with hyperviscosity syndrome and anemia and the conditions that can lead to these hematologic states.

T. Moreno
Florida Retina Institute, Jacksonville, FL, USA

S. J. Kim
Vanderbilt Eye Institute, Nashville, TN, USA

I. U. Scott (✉)
Penn State College of Medicine, Hershey, PA, USA
e-mail: iscott@pennstatehealth.psu.edu

Leukemia

Leukemia is a group of cancers that usually begin in the bone marrow and result in high numbers of abnormal and immature white blood cells, typically called blasts. Systemic symptoms are common but varied and may include bleeding, bruising, fatigue, malaise, fever, and increased risk of infection. The exact cause of leukemia in most cases is unknown, but both inherited and environmental factors are believed to be involved. Known risk factors include smoking, ionizing radiation, chemicals (benzene), prior chemotherapy, Down syndrome, and family history (Hutter 2010). Diagnosis is generally made by blood tests or bone marrow biopsy.

Systemic Classification of Leukemia

Leukemia is a neoplasm of leukocytes and is classified according to its cell of origin, maturity, morphology, and immunophenotype (Mehta et al. 2014). Generally, leukemias are classified into acute or chronic forms as well as lymphoid or myeloid cell types. Acute forms of leukemia are characterized by replacement of the bone marrow with immature white blood cells called blasts and have a more virulent course and must be treated aggressively. Chronic leukemias have a more indolent course and occur from a deregulation of mature leukocytes. Some chronic leukemias do not require prompt treatment but can transform into an aggressive type (blast crisis).

R. V. P. Chan (ed.), *Pediatric Retinal Diseases*, Retina Atlas, https://doi.org/10.1007/978-981-19-1364-8_11

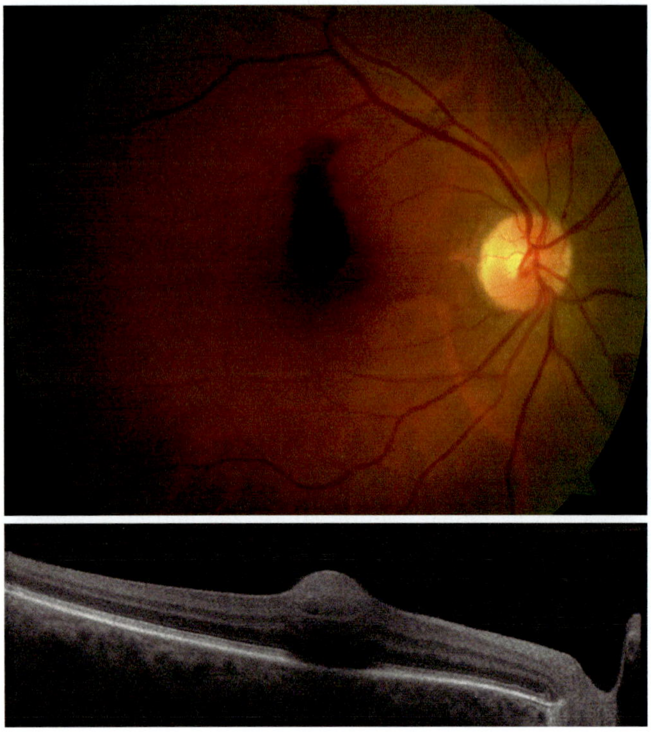

Fig. 11.1 Intraretinal hemorrhage in a patient with acute myeloid leukemia (AML) with concurrent anemia and thrombocytopenia

Epidemiology

The data on the prevalence of ocular involvement in leukemia come from a few prospective studies and autopsy studies and range from 30 to 90%. In a large prospective study of 288 cases of newly diagnosed leukemia, ocular manifestations were present in 35% of affected patients (Reddy et al. 2003). Eye findings were more often observed in adults (49%) than children (17%) and in myeloid leukemia (41%) than lymphoid leukemia (29%). Ocular symptoms were present in 10% of patients. In a recent prospective study of 67 adult patients with leukemia without bone marrow transplant, ocular lesions were found in 52% of patients (Gawai et al. 2016). Ocular involvement was observed more commonly in acute leukemias (63%) than chronic leukemias and in myeloid leukemias (56%) than lymphoid leukemias. Karesh et al. found retinopathy in 53% of patients in a prospective study of 56 patients with previously untreated acute myeloid leukemia (Karesh et al. 1989). Schachat et al. examined 120 patients with newly diagnosed leukemia and found direct leukemic infiltration of the retina in 3% of patients and other ocular findings related to leukemia in 39% of patients (Schachat et al. 1989).

Autopsy series have also shown variable prevalence rates of ocular manifestations among patients with leukemia. An analysis of 135 autopsy eyes found leukemic cell infiltrates in 31% of eyes (Leonardy et al. 1990). The same study found that the prevalence of ocular leukemic cell infiltration tended to gradually decline over time during the study, suggesting that improvements in the treatment of leukemia might be associated with a decrease in the prevalence rate of ocular manifestations. Allen and Straatsma found 50% of cases had ocular involvement, or had pathologic changes which could be directly ascribed to leukemia (Allen and Straatsma 1961). Green and Kincaid reviewed all postmortem eyes obtained at the Wilmer Eye Institute from 1923 to 1980, a total of 383 eyes from patients with leukemia, and found that 82% of patients with acute leukemias and 75% of patients with chronic leukemias had intraocular involvement at the time of death (Kincaid and Green 1983). The choroid was the site most frequently involved histopathologically.

Clinical Features

The retina is the most commonly involved ocular site in clinical studies of leukemia, while the choroid is the most commonly involved ocular site in autopsy studies. Retinal manifestations of leukemia can be divided into direct infiltration by neoplastic cells; secondary or indirect manifestation of leukemia due to anemia, thrombocytopenia, or hyperviscosity; the result of treatment; and the result of opportunistic infections from an immunocompromised state. Secondary manifestations are far more common than primary manifestations.

Direct Retinal Invasion

Direct retinal invasion by neoplastic cells is a rare manifestation of systemic leukemia. Schachat et al. found direct retinal invasion in approximately 3% of patients in a prospective study of 120 patients with leukemia (Schachat et al. 1989). Clinical findings may consist of large gray or white nodules extending into the vitreous often associated with retinal hemorrhage (Kuwabara 1964). Leukemic infiltrates can also be more discrete areas of white infiltrate at the fovea and/or scattered throughout the retina, or present as subretinal hypopyon (Schworm et al. 1995; Le et al. 2016). Perivascular invasion in the retina resembling frosted branch angiitis has also been reported (Kim et al. 1994).

White-centered hemorrhages, or Roth spots, are a common manifestation of leukemia found in 11–25% of patients with leukemia in published clinical trials (Schachat et al. 1989; Gawai et al. 2016). This finding may be the result of leukemic infiltrate (Duane et al. 1980). However, white-centered hemorrhages can also be composed of fibrin and, therefore, may not necessarily be a definite sign of neoplastic invasion.

Choroidal Infiltration

Although the choroid is the most commonly infiltrated ocular structure in leukemia, the clinical findings can be subtle. Exudative retinal detachments or retinal pigment epithelial (RPE) detachments are a hallmark of choroidal infiltration (Kincaid et al. 1979). The fluorescein angiogram can present with a focal area of hyperfluorescence or a more diffuse, "starry night," presentation resembling Vogt–Koyanagi–Harada disease (Sharma et al. 2016). The RPE can have pigmentary changes simulating leopard spots secondary to RPE hypertrophy as a result of leukemic cell infiltration in the retina and choroid (Clayman et al. 1972).

Spectral domain optical coherence tomography (SDOCT) has provided additional insights into the pathophysiology of exudative retinal detachments associated with leukemia. Marked choroidal thickening can be seen by enhanced depth SDOCT in exudative retinal detachments caused by choroidal infiltration of leukemic cells (Adam et al. 2015). These exudative retinal detachments can resolve with chemotherapy treatment and the choroidal thickness may thin to a normal or less than normal thickness (Yalcinbayir et al. 2017).

Vitreous Infiltration

Leukemic infiltration of the vitreous is a rare manifestation of leukemia or leukemia relapse. It can present as dense vitreous cell with or without choroidal or retinal involvement. Aspiration of the vitreous sent for cytology can show leukemic or blast cells, and vitreous infiltration may be the presenting sign of central nervous system (CNS) involvement. Leukemic cells can also enter the vitreous through vitreous hemorrhage if the peripheral blood contains tumor cells. Swartz and Schumann describe a case in which vitreous infiltration was the first sign of relapsing acute lymphoblastic leukemia (Swartz and Schumann 1980). A vitreous sample and lumbar puncture both showed blast cells, while the peripheral blood was negative for malignant cells. The patient was treated with chemotherapy and radiation, and the vitreous infiltration cleared and vision was unaffected (Swartz and Schumann 1980). The leukemic infiltrate may clear with chemotherapy and radiation alone; however, pars plana vitrectomy may also be needed to improve visual acuity in patients with non-clearing vitreous infiltration secondary to leukemia (Zhioua et al. 2001).

Optic Nerve Infiltration

The optic nerve is affected in 2–20% of patients with leukemia. Optic nerve infiltration may present as unilateral or bilateral optic nerve head swelling and can also be associated with vascular complications such as hemorrhage, central retinal artery occlusion, and/or vein occlusion (Salazar Mendez and Fonolla Gil 2014). Manifestations of the optic nerve can be secondary to direct optic nerve head invasion or papilledema secondary to retrolaminar leukemic invasion or increased intracranial pressure (Kincaid et al. 1979). Optic nerve head involvement requires CNS fluid analysis with lumbar puncture(s) to confirm diagnosis and imaging tests. Imaging testing with brain and orbit magnetic resonance imaging (MRI) can determine the extent of optic nerve infiltration and also detect other CNS lesions that may direct treatment (Khan et al. 2016). Most, if not all, patients with optic nerve involvement have CNS involvement. However, the CSF fluid may be negative for neoplastic cells and confirmatory diagnosis has also been obtained by direct optic nerve sheath biopsy (Khan et al. 2016). Patients with optic nerve involvement require prompt treatment and are often treated with a combination of intrathecal and systemic chemotherapy and radiation.

Leukemic Retinopathy

The term leukemic retinopathy often describes the manifestation of anemia, thrombocytopenia, and increased blood viscosity in patients with leukemia. These findings commonly include intraretinal hemorrhages at any layer, white-centered hemorrhages, dilated and tortuous veins, and cotton-wool spots (Reddy et al. 2003). Other less common manifestations of leukemic retinopathy include central retinal vein occlusions (Fig. 11.2), vitreous hemorrhages, localized choroidal hemorrhages, subhyaloid hemorrhages (Fig. 11.3), intraretinal microaneurysms, peripheral retinal neovascularization, and optic nerve head neovascularization (Kincaid and Green 1983; Schachat et al. 1989).

There are conflicting studies with respect to the correlation of retinopathy and the red blood cell count, leukocyte count, and platelet level with many studies not demonstrating a high correlation between retinopathy and blood counts (Kincaid and Green 1983). In a prospective study of 53 patients with leukemia, the presence of retinopathy was

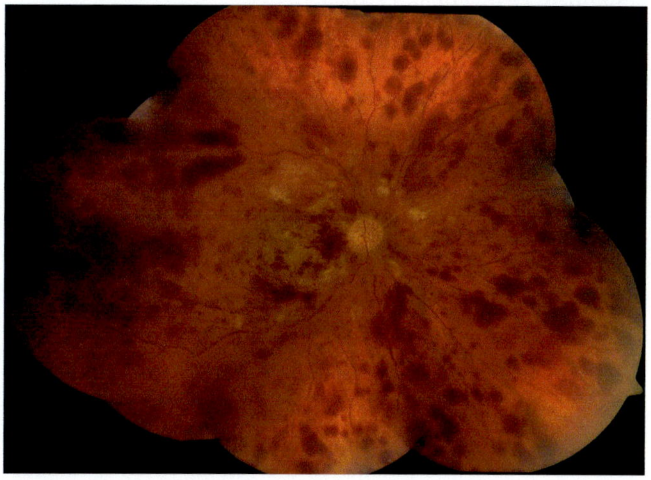

Fig. 11.2 Central retinal vein occlusion in a patient with chronic myeloid leukemia (CML) presenting after recent conversion to blastic phase

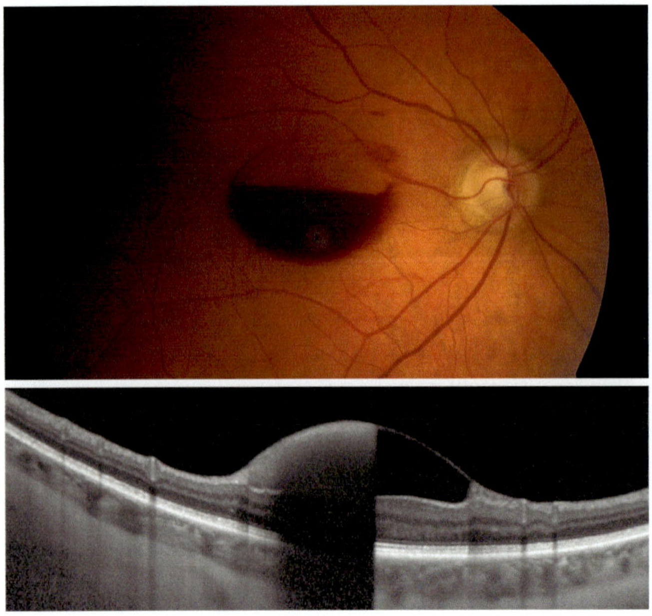

Fig. 11.3 Boat-shaped subhyaloid versus sub-internal limiting membrane hemorrhage in patient with AML with visible fluid level. Vertical optical coherence tomography image demonstrates shadowing effect from coalesced blood and absence of shadowing effect through plasma

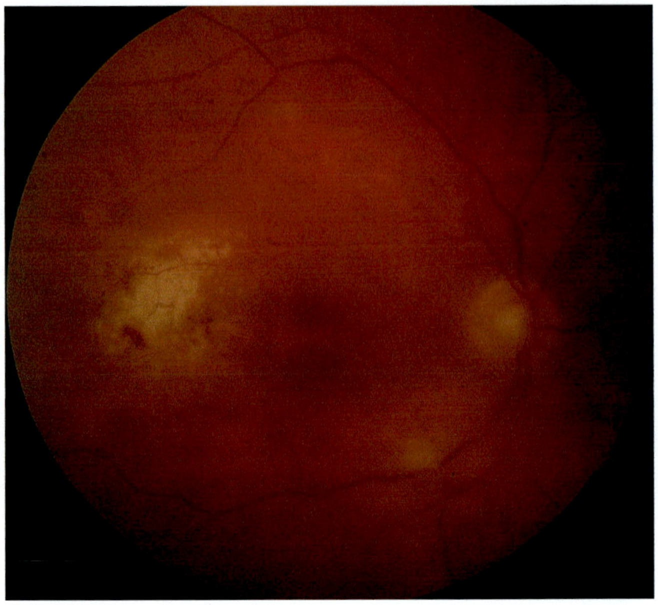

Fig. 11.4 Cytomegalovirus retinitis in a patient undergoing chemotherapy for acute lymphocytic leukemia. Note the predominately non-necrotizing presentation in the macula with central coalesced granular white lesions with associated satellite lesions at the periphery

significantly correlated with platelet count but not with hematocrit or leukocyte count (Karesh et al. 1989). Leonardy et al. reported a significant positive correlation between leukemic cell infiltration of the eye and leukocyte count but found that platelet count was not significantly different in patients with retinal hemorrhages versus those without retinal hemorrhages (Leonardy et al. 1990). It is postulated that the blood profile varies during the course of the disease, and the emergence of the fundus findings may be delayed, correlating better with the blood cell counts of a month or more previously (Kincaid and Green 1983).

Leukemia and Opportunistic Infections

Patients with leukemia are susceptible to life-threatening opportunistic infections that can also manifest with retinal findings. These include infections from viral, fungal, protozoal, and bacterial organisms (Cogan 1977).

Among the viruses, cytomegalovirus (CMV) is one of the most prevalent opportunistic infections (Fig. 11.4). The majority of CMV retinitis is related to hematogenous spread of the virus to the retina, usually after systemic reactivation of latent infection, which may cause retinal necrosis, discrete cream or white patches in the retina, vascular sheathing, hemorrhage, and combined exudative and rhegmatogenous retinal detachments (Meredith et al. 1979). The incidence of CMV retinitis in patients with acute lymphocytic leukemia in maintenance phase of chemotherapy who have not received hematopoietic cell transplantation (HCT) is estimated to be 3.6% (Samia et al. 2014). Other viruses including herpes simplex, varicella zoster, and mumps may also cause necrotizing retinitis in immunocompromised hosts (Cogan 1977). Mumps virus was reported to lead to granulomatous uveitis in a 9-year-old patient with acute lymphocytic leukemia in remission (Al-Rashid and Cress 1977).

Fungi are also common opportunistic infections in patients with leukemia. *Candida Albicans* can present with focal, deep white, choroidal lesions that can extend through Bruch's membrane and the retina into the vitreous as characteristic cotton or snowballs (Cogan 1977). *Aspergillus* can produce more severe intraocular lesions than *Candida* with one or more exudative appearing foci in the choroid with fluffy masses in the vitreous and subsequent retinal detachment (Cogan 1977). Mucor involves the eye more commonly by extension from the orbit and adjacent sinuses. Mucormycosis has been reported to cause bilateral vision loss by invading the optic nerve sheath and optic chiasm in an immunocompromised patient with CML. The patient presented with retinal whitening similar to that of a central retinal artery occlusion and optic nerve pallor (Nerkelun et al. 1997). Nocardia, a gram-positive, weakly acid-fast rod-shaped bacteria, initially misclassified as an aerobic yeast because of its branching filamentary structure, can lead to choroidal abscesses in patients with leukemia (Silva et al. 2015). Prompt awareness, recognition, and treatment of these opportunistic infections may improve prognosis significantly.

Adult T-cell leukemia (ATL) is a malignant lymphoproliferative disorder caused by the retrovirus human T-cell lymphotropic virus type-1 (HTLV-1). Less than 5% of individuals infected by HTLV-1 develop ATL. Retinal manifestations of this condition are rare, but deep retinal infiltrates are the most constant and characteristic finding in ATL-related retinal disease (Merle et al. 2016). Intermediate uveitis is typically seen in patients with retinal involvement but does not aid in the diagnosis as uveitis is frequent among HTLV-1 carriers (Merle et al. 2016). Other retinal manifestations include whitish sheathing of veins and arteries, whitish round-shaped retinal infiltrates that tend to coalesce and progress toward the posterior pole, multiple punctate hyperfluorescent lesions on fluorescein angiography (FA), adjacent remodeled RPE giving the angiographic image of leopard spots, and necrotizing retinal vasculitis (Merle et al. 2016). FA is recommended in all carriers of HTLV-1 with uveitis because deep retinal infiltrates on FA would raise suspicion for ATL (Merle et al. 2016).

Treatment of Leukemia and Retinal Manifestations of Treatment

Treatment of leukemia is evolving rapidly and depends on its classification (acute versus chronic; lymphocytic versus myelodysplastic). While specific details are beyond the scope of this chapter, most treatment protocols use systemic chemotherapy with or without radiotherapy. Intrathecal methotrexate can also be used. Since tumor cells typically divide more rapidly than host cells, chemotherapeutic agents are chosen that interfere with cell division. A combination of vincristine, prednisone, and L-asparaginase is commonly initiated to induce remission for acute lymphocytic leukemia (ALL), while daunorubicin, cytarabine, and thioguanine are commonly used to induce remission in acute myeloid leukemia (AML). In cases where leukocytosis is greater than 100,000 cells, emergent leukapheresis is sometimes necessary to prevent hyperviscosity-related complications. Treatment for both chronic lymphocytic leukemia (CLL) and chronic myeloid leukemia (CML) is often palliative. Treatment for CML is usually initiated when conversion to the blastic phase occurs. Allogeneic bone marrow transplant can be curative for treatment-resistant leukemia, but carries a high risk of early mortality.

As hematological parameters normalize with systemic treatment, many retinal manifestations of leukemia resolve spontaneously. Therefore, ophthalmic treatment of leukemic retinopathy is mainly supportive in nature. When retinal leukemic infiltrates fail to respond to systemic chemotherapy, radiation can be considered. Optic nerve head infiltration requires immediate and prompt intervention, typically with radiation, in order to try to preserve vision.

Treatment of leukemia involves suppression of the host's immune system, which increases the risk of many opportunistic infections. Awareness of this risk, patient education about signs and symptoms, and regular monitoring are necessary for prompt diagnosis and treatment. Common opportunistic infections include herpes-related retinitis, toxoplasma retinochoroiditis, and endogenous fungal endophthalmitis. Delay in a diagnosis of an opportunistic infection can occur if initial manifestation of such an infection is believed to be leukemic retinopathy.

Hyperviscosity Syndromes Other Than Leukemia

Hyperviscosity syndrome (HVS) refers to the clinical sequelae of increased blood viscosity. Increased serum viscosity usually results from increased circulating serum immunoglobulins which can be seen in paraproteinemias such as Waldenstrom macroglobulinemia and multiple myeloma. HVS can also be seen in hyperproliferative states (increased cellular blood components) such as leukemias, myeloproliferative disorders, and polycythemia. Hypercoagulable disease states such as antiphospholipid antibody syndrome and factor V Leiden can also increase blood viscosity. Common retinal findings of HVS (hyperviscosity retinopathy) include retinal vein engorgement, lipid exudates, central and branch retinal vein thrombosis, flame-shaped hemorrhages, cotton wool spots, retinal edema, and, less commonly, serous retinal detachment. In general, treatment of HVS is primarily aimed at the underlying disorder; treatment of retinopathy is mainly supportive. Specific examples are described below.

Paraproteinemias

Waldenstrom macroglobulinemia (WM) is a lymphoproliferative B-cell disorder characterized by overproduction of monoclonal IgM. It is a rare disease with an estimated incidence of three cases per million people per year in the USA which translates into roughly 1000 new diagnoses each year. IgM is a large molecular compound secreted in a pentamer form and mostly contained within the intravascular compartment. IgM can also form aggregates. These attributes contribute to approximately 30–40% of individuals with WM demonstrating some degree of hyperviscosity retinopathy (Orellana and Friedman 1981). Furthermore, recent case studies have associated WM with serous macular detachments presumably from accumulation of IgM in the subretinal space which leads to an increased oncotic gradient causing fluid transudation.

Multiple myeloma (MM) is characterized by proliferation of malignant plasma cells and the subsequent overabundance of monoclonal paraprotein. MM is part of a spectrum of diseases ranging from monoclonal gammopathy of unknown significance (MGUS) to plasma cell leukemia. Osteolytic lesions and pathologic fractures may be seen on skeletal survey. In addition to hyperviscosity retinopathy, other common ocular findings include crystalline keratopathy and ciliary body cysts.

Hyperproliferative States

Polycythemia vera (PV) is caused by neoplastic proliferation of erythroid, megakaryocytic, and granulocytic elements. This results in the overproduction of red blood cells, white blood cells, and platelets. Most of the health concerns associated with PV are due to increased red blood cells. The prevalence of PV is estimated to be 44–57 cases per 100,000 persons; approximately 148,000 persons are living with PV in the USA (Mehta et al. 2014). Treatment can consist of phlebotomy, aspirin, and chemotherapy.

Essential thrombocythemia (ET) is a nonreactive, chronic myeloproliferative disorder in which sustained megakaryocyte proliferation leads to an increase in the number of circulating platelets. It is characterized by a persistently elevated platelet count greater than 450,000/μl. ET is a rare disease with limited prevalence data.

Hypereosinophilic syndrome (HES) is a myeloproliferative disorder characterized by persistently elevated eosinophil count (≥1500 eosinophils/mm^3) in blood for at least 6 months without any recognizable cause and signs and symptoms of organ involvement.

Hypercoagulable States

Protein S deficiency is a disorder mainly associated with increased risk of venous thrombosis. Protein S is a vitamin K-dependent anticoagulant that is a cofactor to activate protein C which, in turn, degrades factors Va and VIIIa. Decreased levels or impaired function of protein S results in decreased degradation of factors Va and VIIIa and increased propensity to venous thrombosis.

Protein C deficiency is associated with increased risk of venous thromboembolism (relative risk 8–10), but no association with arterial thrombotic disease has been shown. Protein C acts as an anticoagulant and inhibits coagulation factors V and VIII.

Antithrombin III (ATIII) is a nonvitamin K-dependent protease that inhibits coagulation by neutralizing the enzymatic activity of thrombin (factors IIa, IXa, Xa). ATIII activity is markedly potentiated by heparin. Deficiency of ATIII increases the risk of venous and arterial thrombosis.

Factor V Leiden is a variant form of human factor V (one of several substances that helps blood clot) which prevents a normally secreted anticoagulant protein from binding to itself and, thus, its presence leads to a hypercoagulable state. Factor V Leiden is the most common hereditary hypercoagulable disorder among ethnic Europeans.

Thrombotic thrombocytopenia purpura (TTP) is a rare blood disorder characterized by extensive microscopic thrombi which form in small vessels resulting in a low platelet count. Most cases of TTP arise from autoantibody-mediated inhibition of the enzyme ADAMTS13, a metalloprotease responsible for cleaving large multimers of von Willebrand factor (vWF) into smaller units. The increase in circulating multimers of vWF increases platelet adhesion to areas of endothelial injury which, in turn, results in formation of thrombi causing microvascular disease.

Disseminated intravascular coagulation (DIC) is characterized by systemic activation of blood coagulation resulting in generation and deposition of fibrin which leads to microvascular thrombi formation in various organs. Because of this, DIC can lead to multiple organ dysfunction syndrome. Consumption and consequent depletion of coagulation proteins and platelets due to ongoing activation of coagulation may induce severe bleeding. Therefore, a patient with DIC can present with simultaneous thrombosis and bleeding which complicates treatment. DIC is most commonly observed in the setting of septic shock and severe sepsis. Purtscher-like retinopathy has been described in cases of DIC.

Antiphospholipid antibody syndrome (APS) is characterized by persistently elevated levels of antibodies directed against membrane anionic phospholipids (i.e., anticardiolipin antibody, antiphosphatidylserine) or their associated plasma proteins (predominately beta-2 glycoprotein 1). APS manifests as recurrent venous or arterial thrombosis and/or fetal loss (Fig. 11.5).

Hyperhomocysteinemia is either due to cystathionine beta-synthase deficiency or from other abnormalities of folate metabolism. Homozygous deficiency of cystathionine beta-synthase can result in plasma homocysteine levels ≥10-fold higher than normal. Milder elevations are seen in heterozygous deficiency or abnormalities of folate metabolism. The most common causes of hyperhomocysteinemia are acquired deficiencies of folate, vitamin B12, and vitamin B6. Hyperhomocysteinemia may predispose to arterial and venous thrombosis due to injury to vascular endothelial cells. Dietary supplementation of folic acid, vitamin B12, and vitamin B6 may normalize levels of homocysteine.

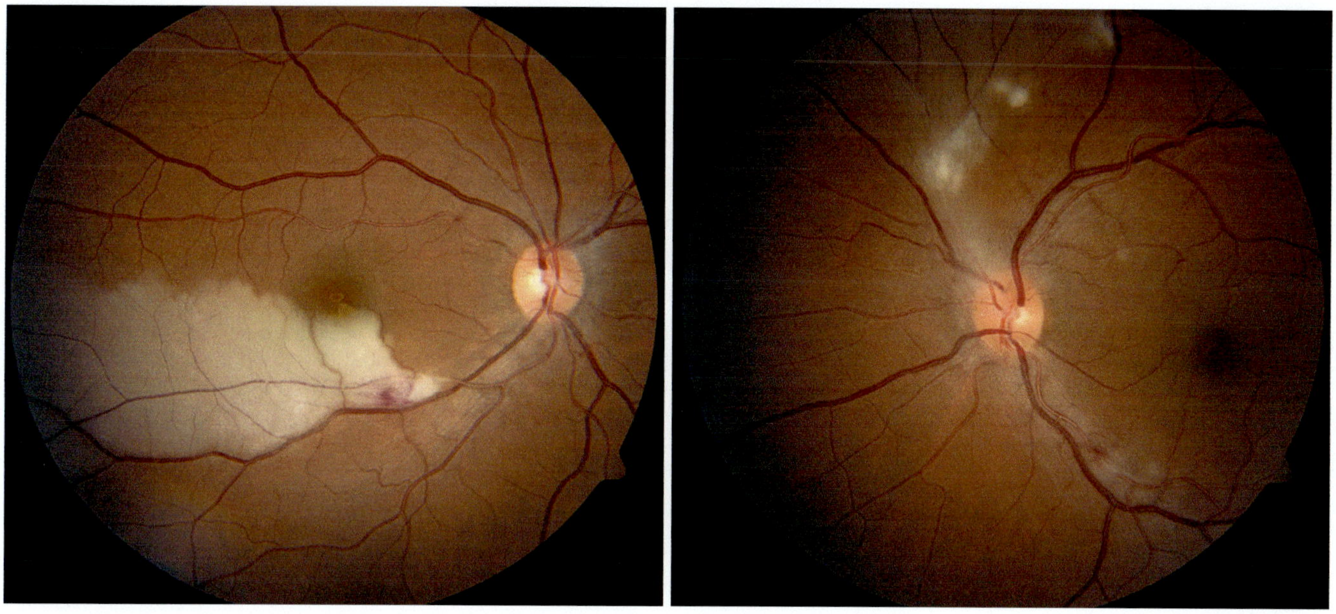

Fig. 11.5 Consecutive bilateral branch retinal artery occlusions in a 28-year-old female, 5 weeks pregnant, with previous history of two miscarriages. Work-up revealed elongated partial thromboplastin time (PTT) and positive lupus anticoagulant consistent with antiphospholipid antibody syndrome

Anemia

Anemia occurs when the level of healthy red blood cells or hemoglobin is too low. Anemia can be due to nutritional deficiency (iron, folate, vitamin B12), blood loss, or inadequate production (aplastic anemia) or increased destruction (hemolytic) of red blood cells. Iron deficiency is the most common type of anemia. A deficiency of vitamin B12 is known as pernicious anemia. Transient retinal hemorrhages in the setting of anemia were first described by Ulrich in 1883 in association with gastrointestinal hemorrhage (Pears and Pickering 1960). Retinopathy in patients with anemia is a common finding, particularly with coexisting thrombocytopenia. Findings include retinal and choroidal hemorrhages, Roth's spots, cotton wool spots, retinal edema, exudates, and venous tortuosity.

A number of factors may contribute to the pathologic changes seen in anemic retinopathy. Retinal hypoxia results in infarction of the nerve fiber layer (cotton wool spots) and may increase VEGF levels, which subsequently increase vascular permeability. Retinal hypoxia also increases vascular dilation and results in both hypoproteinemia (alters transmural oncotic pressure) and microvascular trauma which results in retinal edema and hemorrhage. In many situations, thrombocytopenia occurs concomitantly with anemia and leads to defective coagulation and hemorrhages.

Treatment of the underlying cause of anemia and/or blood transfusions usually addresses the retinopathy.

References

Adam MK, Pitcher JD, Shields CL, Maguire JI. Enhanced depth imaging optical coherence tomography of precursor cell leukemic choroidopathy before and after chemotherapy. Middle East Afr J Ophthalmol. 2015;22(2):249–52.

Allen RA, Straatsma BR. Ocular involvement in leukemia and allied disorders. Arch Ophthalmol. 1961;66:490–508.

Al-Rashid RA, Cress C. Mumps uveitis complicating the course of acute leukemia. J Pediatr Ophthalmol. 1977;14(2):100–2.

Clayman HM, Flynn JT, Koch K, Israel C. Retinal pigment epithelial abnormalities in leukemic disease. Am J Ophthalmol. 1972;74(3):416–9.

Cogan DG. Immunosuppression and eye disease. First Vail lecture. Am J Ophthalmol. 1977;83(6):777–88.

Duane TD, Osher RH, Green WR. White centered hemorrhages: their significance. Ophthalmology. 1980;87(1):66–9.

Gawai D, Jhavar S, Patil S. Orbital and ocular manifestations of acute and chronic leukemia. Int J Health Sci Res. 2016;6(9):61–4.

Hutter JJ. Childhood leukemia. Pediatr Rev. 2010;31(6):234–41.

Karesh JW, Goldman EJ, Reck K, Kelman SE, Lee EJ, Schiffer CA. A prospective ophthalmic evaluation of patients with acute myeloid leukemia: correlation of ocular and hematologic findings. J Clin Oncol. 1989;7(10):1528–32.

Khan K, Malik AI, Almarzouqi SJ, Morgan ML, Yalamanchili S, Chevez-Barrios P, Lee AG. Optic neuropathy due to chronic lymphocytic leukemia proven with optic nerve sheath biopsy. J Neuroophthalmol. 2016;36(1):61–6.

Kim TS, Duker JS, Hedges TR III. Retinal angiopathy resembling unilateral frosted branch angiitis in a patient with relapsing acute lymphoblastic leukemia. Am J Ophthalmol. 1994;117(6):806–8.

Kincaid MC, Green WR. Ocular and orbital involvement in leukemia. Surv Ophthalmol. 1983;27(4):211–32.

Kincaid MC, Green WR, Kelley JS. Acute ocular leukemia. Am J Ophthalmol. 1979;87(5):698–702.

Kuwabara T. Leukemic miliary nodules in the retina. Arch Ophthalmol. 1964;72:494–7.

Le JQ, Braich PS, Brar VS. Optical coherence tomography findings of bilateral foveal leukemic infiltration. Int Med Case Rep J. 2016;9:237–40.

Leonardy NJ, Rupani M, Dent G, Klintworth GK. Analysis of 135 autopsy eyes for ocular involvement in leukemia. Am J Ophthalmol. 1990;109(4):436–44.

Mehta J, Wang H, Iqbal SU, Mesa R. Epidemiology of myeloproliferative neoplasms in the United States. Leuk Lymphoma. 2014;55(3):595–600.

Meredith TA, Aaberg TM, Reeser FH. Rhegmatogenous retinal detachment complicating cytomegalovirus retinitis. Am J Ophthalmol. 1979;87(6):793–6.

Merle H, Hage R, Meniane JC, Deligny C, Plumelle Y, Donnio A, Jean-Charles A. Retinal manifestations in adult T-cell leukemia/lymphoma related to infection by the human T-cell lymphotropic virus type-1. Retina. 2016;36(7):1364–71.

Nerkelun S, Kellermann S, Nenning H. Acute blindness caused by fungal infection in chronic myeloid leukemia. Klin Monatsbl Augenheilkd. 1997;211(4):272–4.

Orellana J, Friedman AH. Ocular manifestations of multiple myeloma, Waldenstrom's macroglobulinemia and benign monoclonal gammopathy. Surv Ophthalmol. 1981;26(3):157–69.

Pears MA, Pickering GW. Changes in the fundus oculi after haemorrhage. Q J Med. 1960;29:153–78.

Reddy SC, Jackson N, Menon BS. Ocular involvement in leukemia–a study of 288 cases. Ophthalmologica. 2003;217(6):441–5.

Salazar Mendez R, Fonolla Gil M. Unilateral optic disk edema with central retinal artery and vein occlusions as the presenting signs of relapse in acute lymphoblastic leukemia. Arch Soc Esp Oftalmol. 2014;89(11):454–8.

Samia L, Hamam R, Dbaibo G, Saab R, El-Solh H, Abboud M, Muwakkit S. Cytomegalovirus retinitis in children and young adults with acute lymphoblastic leukemia in Lebanon. Leuk Lymphoma. 2014;55(8):1918–21.

Schachat AP, Markowitz JA, Guyer DR, Burke PJ, Karp JE, Graham ML. Ophthalmic manifestations of leukemia. Arch Ophthalmol. 1989;107(5):697–700.

Schworm HD, Nasemann JE, Schriever S. Subretinal hypopyon in prolymphocytic leukaemia. Br J Ophthalmol. 1995;79(9):863–4.

Sharma H, Majumder PD, Rao C, Biswas J. A case of acute myeloid leukemia masquerading as unilateral exudative detachment. Am J Ophthalmol Case Rep. 2016;4:47–9.

Silva RA, Young R, Sridhar J, G. Nocardia Study. Nocardia choroidal abscess: risk factors, treatment strategies, and visual outcomes. Retina. 2015;35(10):2137–46.

Swartz M, Schumann GB. Acute leukemic infiltration of the vitreous diagnosed by pars plana aspiration. Am J Ophthalmol. 1980;90(3):326–30.

Yalcinbayir O, Baytan B, Gelisken O, Can B, Sezgin Evim M, Yildiz M, Meral Gunes A. Spectral domain optical coherence tomography findings of patients under treatment for pediatric acute lymphoblastic leukemia. J AAPOS. 2017;21(2):131–135 e131.

Zhioua R, Boussen I, Malek I, Ouertani A. Acute lymphoblastic leukemia and vitreous infiltration. A case study. J Fr Ophtalmol. 2001;24(2):180–2.

MIX
Papier aus verantwortungsvollen Quellen
Paper from responsible sources
FSC® C105338

If you have any concerns about our products,
you can contact us on
ProductSafety@springernature.com

In case Publisher is established outside the EU,
the EU authorized representative is:
Springer Nature Customer Service Center GmbH
Europaplatz 3, 69115 Heidelberg, Germany

Printed by Libri Plureos GmbH
in Hamburg, Germany